Listening
to
Mother

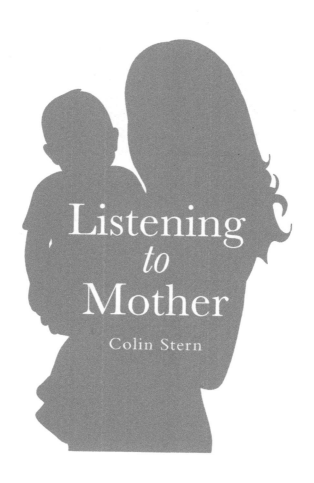

Listening
to
Mother

Colin Stern

BROWN DOG BOOKS

Published under licence by Brown Dog Books and
The Self-Publishing Partnership Ltd, 10b Greenway Farm, Bath Rd, Wick, nr. Bath BS30 5RL

www.selfpublishingpartnership.co.uk

ISBN paperback book: 978-1-83952-350-2
ISBN hardback book: 978-1-83952-351-9
ISBN e-book: 978-1-83952-352-6

Cover design by Kevin Rylands
Internal design by Andrew Easton

Printed and bound in the UK
This book is printed on FSC certified paper

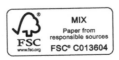

MIX
Paper from
responsible sources
FSC
www.fsc.org
FSC® C013604

Contents

Introduction

I've been so lucky. Working with children was a joy. I have often told friends that I had the best clinical job in London. When I qualified and started my training, we worked ridiculous hours. During one six-month post I left the hospital only once, for a day. When I became a Postgraduate Dean, I campaigned hard for reductions in the hours spent on call.

However, to be honest, I loved every minute of it. Nowadays people forget that we worked in close-knit teams. We learned from each other. Because we worked for longer, we saw our cases through. Today, that's more difficult to do. There were fewer of us, so we saw a lot more cases. All of this was of enormous benefit to us as clinicians.

I owe my career primarily to three teachers. Dr Philip Evans, a clinician of unsurpassed skill, Professor Peter Tizard, a brilliant man manager and Professor John Davis, once addressed by Prince Philip, 'I believe you're the cleverest paediatrician in Britain.' He was.

My saving graces, once I became a consultant, were two. I had a lot of experience and I was surrounded by a brilliant team. I remember asking a student for his opinions about a case. He asked me in return what I thought he could contribute. I told him that everyone knows things that I don't and, if I don't ask, I'll never discover what they are.

A grandchild said to me a few years ago, 'Grandfather, you're so wise!'. I told him, 'It's a funny thing. The older I get, the more I realise how little I actually do know.' If the cases make me seem clever, remember that I'm describing mostly my successes. It's an illusion.

The cases described in this book are fictional. All the clinical problems actually happened, but I have manipulated them, sufficiently I hope, to make the sources from which I have put them together completely anonymous. The families, their occupations and their locations are all invented.

In writing the book, my intention has been to entertain, to inform and sometimes to amuse or to sadden you, the public. If I have failed, I'm sorry. At least I tried.

1.

Seeing if Daydreaming Fits

One has always to have an open mind when you first meet a family. The Hammonds made an appointment and brought their GP's letter with them, so I had no idea what to expect.

HARRY
'He doesn't look at me!'

Juliet Hammond sat beside her husband, David. They both looked tense and she looked at me anxiously. Harry, their six-week-old baby, snuggled in her arms. He slept peacefully, wrapped in a shawl that I thought might be made of antique cream-coloured Brussels lace. Juliet had fair shoulder-length hair, blue eyes and fine, clear features. She wore a Givenchy black silk trouser suit with a white blouse. David's hands were never still, fiddling with the cuffs of his shirt. He had that bright, clean skin brought about by compulsory cold showers at boarding school. His nose was of City proportions and his fine brown hair, thinning at the forehead, was swept back. He leaned back in his chair, from time to time running a hand over his perspiring brow.

'We think he might be blind,' he said, bluntly.

How long had they been in this state, I asked myself? Clearly social class one and with access to Harley Street, why were they in my NHS clinic? How many private opinions had they sought? I read again the letter they had brought from their private GP.

'Dear doctor,' – obviously not bothered about who they saw, I thought – 'Harry's young parents are extremely anxious about him, having become convinced that he is blind. As he is only one month old, I explained that I could not be sure whether this was so, but that it seemed unlikely to me. Mrs Hammond says that Harry does not look at her when she feeds him, or at her husband when he is in the nursery. She has seen other babies of the same age who do watch their mothers. I have been unable to reassure them and I hope that you will be able to do so.'

This sort of letter tends to make me feel uneasy. The GP sounded irritated by the Hammonds and not very tolerant of their anxiety. It would have been easy to convey this sort of impatience to the parents, which would not have helped the situation. Even if there were nothing wrong with Harry, it would be important to show them that all was well. Their doctor didn't seem to be aware that it is easy to show whether a baby can see, even when they are newborn. I turned back to the Hammonds.

'Well,' I said vaguely, 'You say that Harry doesn't look at you. Would you like to tell me about it?'

'I know we are being silly about this,' Juliet Hammond said, 'and we apologise for wasting your time ...'

Help! This is always a bad sign. When parents start to apologise as soon as we meet, I know that someone, somewhere has told them, brusquely and in no uncertain terms; that there is nothing wrong with their child and they shouldn't have bothered him with what was so obviously a trivial problem. The flavour of the letter was confirmed.

In one way, these clues often help me to decide which approach will be the most productive. No one had, so far, managed to reassure Mr and Mrs Hammond that Harry had normal vision and being ticked off by a previous doctor would make them defensive about the reasons for their anxiety. I needed to draw these worries out and discover the reasons behind them.

Meanwhile, Juliet continued.

'I don't think Harry can see properly. When I feed or cuddle him, he doesn't seem to look at me. When David plays with him, he seems to be in a daze.' She paused briefly. 'I'm sure he's blind!' she blurted out and a few tears collected in the corners of her eyes and trickled down her cheeks.

'He looks a lovely baby to me,' I said, after giving her a moment to collect herself. 'Why don't you let me hold him for a bit?'

She smiled wanly, and David patted her ineffectively on the shoulder.

Normally, at this point I would have spent more time extracting the minutiae of the clinical history, but it is always better to shape the consultation to the case. The Hammonds were in a state of acute emotional distress. I had been watching Harry's face carefully while Juliet poured out her worries about him. It was time to give them relief.

I took Harry from her arms and walked across to the open doorway of an unlit examination side room and stood with my back to it, facing the bright lights of the clinic.

'Come over here and stand behind me,' I asked.

They did so. I held Harry, who was by now wide awake, up in front of me and at his arm's length. I waited until I knew his eyes were fixed on my face. He opened his mouth and began to push his tongue out at me; a proto-smile. I moved him to the right while I leaned to the left, slowly, and then back again.

'If you watch his face, you can tell that Harry is looking at me. He has focussed his eyes on my face, which is brightly lit against the dark background of the doorway. As I move to the left and the right, you can see that he continues to watch me intently all the time. All babies choose to look at faces rather than objects. You do need to make sure that he has caught sight of you first, as they can't focus very well until around this age. That's why, for younger babies, you need to be about 35 centimetres away. Anyway, there's no doubt that Harry can see quite normally for a baby of his age.'

I heard a faint giggle behind me. They were convinced. As I turned round to hand Harry back to Juliet Hammond, I saw that they had put an arm around each other and were clinging together in their relief.

I had been able to take this short cut, because I had noticed that Harry had woken up and had been watching his mother's face while we were sitting and talking. He had shown none of the wandering eye movements that are typically seen in blind babies. I walked back to my seat.

'Come and sit down. Well, there is no doubt that he can see perfectly well,' I said. 'Just so that I can satisfy my own curiosity, let me ask you a few routine questions about him and then I'll carry out a formal clinical examination, just to make sure.'

I took a history. Juliet said, 'We wanted to be certain that Harry's eyes would be safe when he was born, so we were careful not to expose him to strong light.'

'Was there any special reason for you to believe that Harry's eye might be more sensitive than normal?' I asked.

'Well,' she began to explain, 'I'm the youngest of four children and I was brought up in the ancestral pile in Suffolk. Mummy and Daddy led a rather hectic social life, so the four of us were brought up by a succession of redoubtable Norland nannies, all managed by Grandmamma. She is an Institution and pretty formidable herself, though she adored all of us. She organised our early education, before we went off to boarding school, and checked that our tutor was doing his job properly.' Juliet laughed. 'Grandmamma regaled us with lurid tales of the family, going back hundreds of years. It seems that a number of them were blind, one or two born so, but mostly as a consequence of some accident or illness, all unconnected. Anyway, when a new baby is born into the family, we always take precautions, just in case.'

She smiled at David. 'After university, I went to work at Sotheby's and that's where David and I met. We married two years ago and Harry is the first baby to be born into the family for twenty-five or so. I was the last. We bought this lovely apartment in Bayswater. We've made sure that, sticking to the family's advice, the curtains in Harry's bedroom are drawn for the first few weeks and we haven't taken him out, except to the doctor's and here, and I use a little blindfold for those trips.' She took out a small black eyeshade, of the sort handed out on long haul flights.

All was now clear. Harry wasn't watching Juliet or David because he couldn't see them well enough. The room was too dark.

Harry was becoming restless. 'It's time for his next feed. Do you mind if I start him now?'

'Not at all,' I said. Unselfconsciously, Juliet began to breastfeed him. 'All you need to do is to take him home and open the curtains,' I assured them. 'Soon he will be watching you all the time. I don't think I need to see him again, though.'

'Oh,' David interjected. 'Please would you review him in six months or so?' he asked.

This is sometimes a problem. A review wasn't indicated from a clinical point of view, but this consultation was all about reassurance.

'All right,' I conceded weakly, 'I'll see you in the spring.'

Six months later Juliet, David and Harry returned to my follow-up clinic. Harry was smiling and laughing. He played with his baby toys and did everything he was supposed to do at his age.

'He's wonderful,' I said, enthusiastically. 'There's absolutely nothing wrong with him. Take him home and, if you want me to review him again because of some new problem, please give my secretary a ring.'

This is always a good move, for two reasons. First of all,

I had a marvellous secretary, Gill. We worked together for twenty-six years and she was wonderful at dealing with parents. Secondly, knowing that they could come back if they want to is always reassuring for parents and, with their immediate worries removed, they don't usually return.

'Please could we bring him back at a year?' said Julia. 'Grandmamma says that, if everything fine then, there won't be a problem.'

'Far be it from me to go against her great experience,' I said, ironically. 'I'll see him for one last visit in another six months.'

Harry returned to my clinic with his father. By this time, he was fourteen months old, toddling on his own and spent his first few minutes in the clinic investigating the box of toys on the play mat.

'Hello,' I said. 'Harry looks well and so do you. How is your wife?'

There was a pause.

'I thought you might know,' he said. 'She stopped at the lights and a lorry smashed into the back of her little car. The back of her head was injured and her optical cerebral cortex has gone. She's blind.'

SARAH

Sarah's parents were not in a good frame of mind. Their three-year-old daughter had been referred to me because they were worried about her vision.

Mrs Sands came in holding Sarah's hand. She sat down and Sarah went straight for the toys, picking up a rag doll. She was a pretty, blue-eyed girl in a smocked dress and sat, cross-legged, on the mat.

'Her eyes wander about,' her mother told me. She was an anxious-looking lady with fading blonde hair. Mr Sands was a bluff, hearty chap with a bristly moustache. He left the consultation to his wife, but they held hands for comfort. 'We think her eyesight isn't very good.' Suddenly, she turned on me. 'And it's all the fault of the maternity unit here!' she expostulated.

'Tell me about it,' I replied.

'After she was born, she developed jaundice. They shone lights on her for three days. I'm sure that damaged her eyes, it was so bright.'

Jaundice in newborn babies is common. Babies have a high haemoglobin level when they are born and have a particular form of the molecule that hangs on to oxygen better. They need this because the level of oxygen reaching them across the placenta is low. After birth, haemoglobin falls and converts slowly to its normal type. The breaking down of haemoglobin releases bilirubin, which makes babies turn yellow in their first few days of life. This molecule isn't soluble in water until it has been 'conjugated' by the liver so that it can be excreted, but the enzymes in a baby's liver that do this have to be stimulated by a rise in bilirubin to reach an efficient level. Consequently, babies become jaundiced for a few days until the enzymes are working effectively.

Jean Ward, a sister at Rochford Hospital in Essex in the 1950s, believed that fresh air and sunshine was good for newborn infants. She took them into the fresh air and sunshine regularly, bringing them in when the doctors came round. One of the team, Dr Dodds, observed that a baby under her care had a triangle of deeper yellow on his skin. It transpired that he had been left on a balcony in the sun in a nappy and a sheet corner had been lying across his tummy. Later, the local chemical pathologist, Dr Perryman, discovered that samples of jaundiced blood, left in the sun, turned greenish. Eventually, between them, they realised that, somehow, the sun had bleached the jaundice from the skin. Subsequent research showed that sunlight broke the bilirubin molecule, making it more water-soluble and, therefore, excretable. Since then it has been standard practice to shine light of the appropriate wavelength on babies whose jaundice has risen to an unacceptable level.

There is no evidence that these lights damage babies when used appropriately and, in this case, are not harmful to the eye. In Sarah's case, I needed more information before I said anything that might risk damaging my relationship with the family.

I took a full history, but there was nothing of especial significance in it. However, while I was listening to Mrs Sands, I was watching Sarah, because one can often uncover the cause of a problem before one actually gets to examine a child formally.

Sarah was playing with the clinic toys. She had light brown hair, but there was a flash of white hair just above her forehead; small but distinct. Secondly, I noticed that she would shake her head very slightly and intermittently. I could see that, from time to time, her eyes would move right and left rapidly. although briefly.

By now, I suspected that I knew what the problem might be. There is a group of conditions know as Partial Oculocutaneous Albinism in which there is an impairment of the ability to metabolise tyrosine, an amino-acid. There are several genes responsible for varieties of the condition.

I asked Mrs Sands to sit Sarah on her knee and began my examination. As we progressed, I pointed out the key abnormalities.

'This is interesting,' I said, as I pointed out the white lock of hair.

'Yes,' said Mrs Sands, 'My mother said that there are other relatives that had this, but I can't remember who.'

'It's what we call a "white forelock,"' I said.

As I continued, I noticed that Sarah had several small patches of depigmented skin and demonstrated them.

Because of her intermittent rapid eye movement, and also because she was three, it was hard to get a good view of Sarah's retinae, but I pointed out to the Sands her head shaking and eye movements.

'Putting all these together,' I said, 'I think Sarah has a condition that makes it hard for her to make some chemicals that she needs for normal eyesight. She is getting round the problem by moving her head and her eyes, as this probably helps her to see things more clearly. The condition is called Partial Oculocutaneous Albinism and there are several different forms of it; none of them are very common. We need to ask two of my colleagues here to see her: an children's eye specialist to check her eyes more thoroughly than I can, and a clinical geneticist, who will be able to work out exactly which form of the condition Sarah has.'

I needed to make sure I limited the distress this diagnosis would cause Mr and Mrs Sands.

'Sarah will be fine. Doing these things will help us to help her lead a normal life. One thing I can say for certain: the light treatment didn't affect her at all, which is good. It's a condition that we can help you to manage so Sarah can enjoy life to the full.'

The Sands looked at me doubtfully. 'How can you be sure?' said Mrs Sands.

'One can never be certain of anything,' I replied. 'But this is a condition that I have seen before and I think the clinical signs that we have looked at together fit. I am as sure as one can be that this is the cause of the problem.'

They relaxed. I made arrangements for Sarah's investigations and further consultations, including one with another colleague with a special interest in metabolic disorders.

'I think it best for Sarah to be seen in a special clinic for these sorts of condition,' I explained. 'She doesn't need to see me again, though, if you would like to, here is my secretary's number.'

The diagnosis turned out to be correct. I never saw her again.

BILLY

Billy was a busy boy of eight. He came rushing into the clinic, followed by his parents, who seemed slightly embarrassed by his exuberance. Whatever the problem might be, it hadn't affected his personality.

Mr and Mrs Salmon sat down. Roger Salmon wore a business suit. He worked in a bank. His pretty wife Valerie was worried, but had the strength of character not to show it.

'How can I help?' I asked. Of course, I knew what the problem was from the GP referral letter. Billy's right eye had developed a recent squint and also seemed to be slightly out of position.

'It all happened over the last week or two,' Mrs Salmon said. 'I noticed it when he came down to breakfast last Thursday week. I asked if he was all right and Billy said he was fine. Then over the next few days it didn't get any better. In fact, I think it's a bit worse, although it doesn't seem to have affected him at all.' Billy was busy kicking a small football again a clinic wall. 'Billy, stop that!' she said.

'It's all right,' I said. 'There are very few limits in here!'

I went through the history, but there was nothing else of importance. I called Billy over to be examined. The abnormality of his eye was clear.

His right eye was bulging outward slightly in comparison with his left. The pupil of the right was deviated a little downwards and to the right, causing a squint. Professionally, we would say that he had right-sided mild exophthalmos with external strabismus. With such a short history in a child of this age, who was otherwise in very good health, there was one likely diagnosis. A rhabdomyosarcoma of one of the muscles of the eye. This is a cancer, but, in this position, one with a good prognosis, provided one acts quickly. It was important to let Mr and Mrs Salmon know as gently as possibly.

'You can see that Billy's eye has been slightly displaced. The likely reason is that there is something at the back of his eye that is causing it. The eye sits in a bony shell, so, if something at the back of the eye grows, it will push it forward. I think that is what is happening here. Various things can do this, but the most likely in someone of Billy's age is a tumour.'

His parents flinched, but continued to listen fairly calmly.

'The good thing about this is that, in this position, tumours present very early. The result is that we can deal with them quickly and in virtually all cases the outcome is complete cure.'

They relaxed.

'However, we need to act fast.'

I spent a few more minutes reassuring them and then picked up the telephone. A paediatric ophthalmic surgical colleague saw him that morning and a paediatric oncologist in the afternoon.

Billy had his eye operation within a day or two. As is often the case, the tumour had spread to involve the eye itself very slightly, but this meant that his eye had to be removed. Initially, this was the cause of considerable distress to the family, although not to Billy, whose extrovert personality seemed completely unaffected by this setback.

Billy used to come back to see me from time to time. He had a wonderful childhood, throwing himself into every activity he could find. He became an excellent footballer, though he preferred to play on the right, because 'It's easier to see things on my left!'

His favourite joke when he came to the clinic involved the students, who he loved to tease. He was given a series of glass eyes, which were changed every now and then for a larger size, so that his right orbit would grow to match that on the left.

At some point in the consultation, he would suddenly smack his forehead with his left hand, this caused his glass eye to pop out and roll across the floor. He delighted in the shocked and startled exclamations from the students and then picked up his eye, gave it a quick wipe and popped it back. Irrepressible.

JOANNA

Joanna was twelve years old. According to the letter from her GP, she had been suffering from epilepsy for about four years. Her care had been managed by a paediatrician at her local hospital in the Midlands, but control of her seizures had been becoming less effective as she grew older. The opinion was that this poorer control was the result of the onset of puberty.

The family, consisting of Joanna, her brother James, who was ten, and her parents, David and Olivia Thomas, had recently moved to London, so her care needed to be transferred. Usually, I would have expected Joanna to be seen by a paediatric neurology colleague, but her new family doctor, with whom I had a good relationship, asked me to review her care first. David was an engineer and his wife had been a secretary, but was now a full-time mother.

I shook hands with Joanna and her family and they sat down. James was reading a comic.

'How are you?' I asked.

'Not so good,' Joanna answered. 'I'm still having seizures from time to time, in fact most days.'

'When are they most likely to happen?'

'Quite often when I wake up, or if I'm late going to bed. They happen during the day at odd times. In boring lessons sometimes!'

We all laughed.

I asked about her birth and when her convulsions had started. She was eight when she had her first seizure, which was a generalised one, involving jerking of her arms and legs: a typical grand mal convulsion. She had been investigated and her electroencephalogram (EEG) showed typical spike/wave complexes that affected her motor cortex, together some other abnormalities typical of generalised epilepsy. Her initial treatment had been a drug called phenytoin, which had worked quite well. This drug has been around for a long time and, while today it isn't so much used in children in the UK, having been superseded by better ones, it is still commonly taken in the USA.

'After a while,' said her mother, 'Joanna's seizures returned. They upped her phenytoin dose and, when that didn't work, added carbamazepine and they stopped again. Then more convulsions came back and, after playing around with the doses, they added sodium valproate and they stopped again. After a while, Joanna began to have seizures on getting up and when she was tired, so they added a small dose of clonazepam just before bedtime, to see whether this would help. It hasn't made much difference, but this was only given just before we moved to London.'

'Gosh,' I said to Joanna. 'That's a lot of medicines for you to have to take!'

'It's all right,' she said stoically. 'Well, I wouldn't mind if they actually worked!'

'Her paediatrician said, last time we saw him, that the best way forward might be for Joanna to have brain surgery. He showed some reports where it had been very successful in controlling difficult epilepsy. We weren't at all keen on that!' said Mrs Thomas.

'I think there might be some other possibilities to explore first,' I said.

I finished taking Joanna's history and carried out a thorough clinical examination, focussing on her central nervous system. I didn't find anything abnormal.

I knew that the consultant caring for Joanna up until now was a general paediatrician, like me, not specialised in neurology. I knew also that this was more anti-convulsant medication than was likely to be necessary. Quite often these drugs interact, so that, far from reducing the convulsions a child is having, they may actually be increased. The more different drugs a child takes, the more likely this is to happen. As the medicines affect the electrical impulses in the brain by different mechanisms, it isn't very surprising.

'I think it would be a good moment to reassess Joanna's epilepsy,' I said. 'I think we should repeat her EEG and also perform an MRI (magnetic resonance image) of her brain. We'll check some blood chemistry and also the levels of the medicines in her blood. On a positive note, I think we ought to sit down and work out some changes in her regime. I suspect that we can make it a lot simpler and I have an idea that we should be able to stop Joanna's seizures completely.'

Joanna looked delighted and so did her parents, but a little puzzled.

'How can you do that?' Mrs Thomas asked me.

'Well,' I procrastinated, not wanting to be critical of her present treatment. 'It's possible that some of the medicines don't suit Joanna. By simplifying things, we can sort this out and discover which medicines work best for her. I hope that it won't be a complicated process.'

I was being economical with the truth here. I was certain that the lack of seizure control was due to her being given too many drugs, what we call polytherapy. This is a known cause of the failure of treatment in cases like Joanna's. While I fully intended to transfer her care to the paediatric epilepsy team, I knew this would take a few weeks and I saw no reason to delay.

Joanna, her parents and I got together around my desk and I wrote out a protocol in which we would gradually reduce Joanna's drugs, starting with the clonazepam, then the phenytoin and finally the carbamazepine: these are the drugs that are most likely to cause side effects. At the same time, we would both slowly increase her dose of sodium valproate, as her dose was rather low, and also change her to a slow release formulation, called Epilim Chrono, which would make it easier to prevent her seizures over a twenty-four-hour period.

I arranged to see Joanna at fairly frequent intervals during this process. After they had all left my clinic, taking the forms for Joanna's investigations with them, I wrote a referral to the children's epilepsy clinic.

Joanna made very good progress, about halfway through her treatment changes, her seizures reduced dramatically and once only on Epilim Chrono, they stopped. Her blood levels of valproate were in the therapeutically effective range.

At this point she was seen in the children's epilepsy clinic.

'I don't know why you asked me to see her,' my colleague complained. 'There's nothing for me to do! All her investigations have been done and her epilepsy is well controlled now.'

'I know,' I apologised. 'I didn't want her to have to wait to see you before she was better controlled, so I thought I would just get on with it. Anyway, you can manage her ongoing care much better than I.'

Mollified, he agreed.

MOHAMMED

It's often contentious as to whether a child has had a seizure, or whether it was some other symptom, such as a rigor, which is a shivering attack, often quite brief, associated with a high temperature. This can be particularly complex, as younger children may have convulsions associated with fever, known as febrile seizures. You can imagine the confusion that this can lead to, amongst doctors as well as parents.

Mohammed's case was a little different. His family was from a black African Muslim society, originally from Malawi, who had arrived in Britain about two years before I met him. This nine-month-old boy had been admitted as an emergency though our Children's Accident and Emergency Department, having suffered several seizures at home. His parents had brought him to the hospital, because they were having difficulty accessing a home visit from their family doctor, possibly because his mother spoke no English. Mohammed's father spoke reasonable English and also some Arabic.

The A&E paediatric team had assessed Mohammed as suffering from infantile epilepsy, of which there are many types, from benign to serious or fatal conditions. He had been given a single dose of clonazepam to tide him over the rest of the night, having arrived at 11 pm the previous day.

I came to see him the next morning, on my regular ward round. The Senior House Officer (SHO) had already taken a very full history and examined him, without finding any specific abnormality. He had arranged also a number of investigations, but blood samples had not yet been taken, other than the basic ones taken in A&E, which included a blood culture, although there was nothing to suggest an infection. My Senior Registrar (SR), Dr Elliott, was keen to perform a lumbar puncture, before giving him any more treatment. I spent a few minutes reading his notes.

'Let's just think about this for a moment,' I said. We had the record from his birth, as he had been born at our hospital.

'When you took him home,' I asked through Mohammed's father, 'Was he a healthy baby? Did he take his feeds well?'

'Oh yes,' he replied, after speaking with his wife. 'Very well.'

'Did your wife feed him herself?'

'Oh yes.'

'When did she start to give him food other than breast milk?'

A long discussion followed between husband and wife. There was much nodding and shaking of heads and a flood of what I presumed to be Chewa from Mohammed's mother.

'Well, in our culture we don't start solid food until babies are older,' father said. 'He won't do that until he passes a year of age.'

'I see.'

I had a suspicion about what might be going on here.

'Do you take him out for walks in a pram or a pushchair?'

'Oh no,' said dad, obviously rather horrified. 'When babies are small, they stay inside the house with their mothers.'

'Does your wife go out, perhaps shopping?'

'No,' said Dad firmly. 'My wife's sister does the shopping. My wife had only been outside our house to come to the hospital since Mohammed was born.'

I asked him about the diet that they ate at home, which was much like the food they ate in Malawi. They bought basic foodstuffs and made their meals from scratch. Their basic diet was nsima, a sort of porridge made from pounded maize. They added vegetables to that and also ate fruit.

'Before you came to England, did your wife spend much time outdoors?'

'No,' he said. 'It wasn't safe where we lived. There was a lot of violence, so my wife stayed in the house, where she could be safe.'

I began to examine Mohammed. Before doing anything else, I tapped his right cheekbone gently. The muscles of his face on that side twitched. I did it again. They twitched again. I didn't really need to do anything else, but I completed a quick examination and turned to the SHO and SR.

'Please chase up Mohammed's serum calcium levels and obtain blood from his mother to check her levels too.'

I turned back to Mohammed's father.

'The jerking episodes that Mohammed has been having are not signs that there is anything wrong with his brain. The levels of a blood chemical called calcium are too low. This makes his muscles twitch intermittently and repeatedly and causes an appearance that looks like a seizure. I suspect that your wife's levels may also be low.'

'Why?' he asked.

'For two reasons,' I answered. 'One thing is that the food you eat is low in calcium. The other is that neither your wife, nor your son, have been in the sun. Sunlight is important for health, as it helps your skin to make vitamin D, which is important is controlling the calcium in your body. If the tests show that this is the problem, we can deal with it easily. We can give both your wife and your son extra calcium in their diet and also make sure they get vitamin D as well. Everything will be fine. It is safe for your wife to take Mohammed out on a sunny day though, if you can.'

Eventually, all the tests came back and showed that hypocalcaemia was present both in mother and infant. X-rays showed that both had poor development of their bones as well. After a few months of treatment, Mohammed and his mother were healthy again, and he didn't have any more convulsions.

Dr Elliott said later that she suspected that Mohammed had rickets.

I said, 'Well, there were changes in his epiphyses and metaphyses (at the end of his long bones) that looked suspiciously like those of rickets. I think it was the hypocalcaemic seizures that meant he presented before the rickets had fully developed.'

'Why do you think he presented like this?' she asked.

'Because mum has probably had low calcium levels for a long time, throughout her pregnancy anyway. As a result, Mohammed's total body calcium would have been lower than normal at birth, I think, the basis of his seizures.'

GERALDINE

Sometimes the reasons for a problem are not obvious.

I was asked to see ten-year-old Geraldine Painter by her family doctor in Kent. She had been born in a local hospital and, after a difficult delivery complicated by a period when she was short of oxygen, spent a week or so in their Special Care Baby Unit. She didn't need much supportive treatment and went home, feeding well. After a few months, having been followed up carefully by the community paediatricians, she was discharged.

Her physical development was a little slower than normal. She said her first words at fifteen months and walked at twenty-two months, late but just about within normal limits. She grew normally and went to school when she was rising five years old.

Initially she did well at school and really enjoyed it, making lots of friends. She wasn't especially good at sport, but liked swimming. When she was nine years old, her academic progress slowed. Now, eighteen months later, she was struggling. The reason for her referral was to ask whether I could discover why her school progress has slowed.

'It's really a bit of a puzzle,' said Susan Painter, Geraldine's mother. 'Geraldine was doing really well at school to start with; now she is having trouble keeping up.' She was a harassed-looking mother with hair that flew in all directions. While she was finding the consultation tricky, Geraldine was really in control.

'What do you think is making it difficult for you?' I asked Geraldine.

'I'm not sure really,' she replied. 'I seem to miss out on quite a lot of what my teachers are saying to me, but I'm not sure why. If they sit down and go through it, I can usually get the hang of it. But when I am doing work they have set for me I often don't finish it.'

'Her teachers say that she daydreams and doesn't pay attention in the way that she used to.'

'I try,' said Geraldine, rather indignantly. 'I just don't seem to be able to keep up.'

'Well,' I said, 'let's not get ahead of ourselves. I think I should get a bit more of the story from you and then have a look at you.'

'Okay,' said Geraldine.

I completed the rest of her history and started to have a look at her. Everything was normal until I examined her central nervous system.

The first thing I noticed was that her gait was more widely

based I than expected. I asked her walk on the outside of her feet. She gave me a quizzical look, but complied. When she walked like this, she flexed her right elbow slightly and pronated (turned inwards) her right hand. Seeing this, I asked her to stretch her arms out in front of her with her fingers spread. Then I asked her to pretend to play the piano with each hand independently. She could do this with her left hand, but when she tried to do so with her right hand, her the fingers of her left hand moved as well.

'I can't seem to stop that,' she said.

Although she was right-handed, that hand was slightly smaller than the left hand. When I examined the muscle tone of her arms and legs, the muscle tone seemed to me to be slightly increased and her tendon reflexes were also a bit brisk. The plantar reflex in her right foot was extensor: her big toe went up when I stroked the sole of her foot.

'I know that Geraldine had quite a difficult time as a newborn baby. Your local paediatricians said that she was normal when they discharged her, is that right?'

'Yes,' said Mrs Painter, 'but that was when she was quite small. We haven't seen one since she was two or three years old.'

'Well,' I said, 'I think that Geraldine has some clinical signs that show that her difficult time at birth has had an effect on the way her brain controls her muscles. There is evidence of some damage, although it's clear that she has managed very well since then, so it hasn't caused her any major problems.'

'Could it have anything to do with her problems at school?'

'It might, but we'll need to do some tests to see whether that's the case.'

I arranged for Geraldine to have several investigations, including an MRI scan of her brain and an electroencephalogram (EEG).

When the results were back, I met the Painters again in my clinic. First of all, I showed them her MRI scan.

'I think you can see that the right side of her brain is a little smaller than the left. In addition, there are some tiny little bright areas (I pointed them out). We think these are little scars, left after Geraldine's difficult birth.'

'What does that mean?' Susan Painter asked.

'Just that she had a small amount of brain damage during her birth. It'll make more sense when we look at her EEG report.'

There is never much point in showing the actual test sheets to parents, although I always did, if they asked to see it. To them, it would look like eight to twelve parallel squiggly lines across a lot of paper.

'This report shows that sometimes Geraldine has abnormal electrical activity that particularly affects her parietal cortex.' I pointed out the place on her MRI scan. 'This means that she is having seizures from time to time, although no one would have been aware of them, because Geraldine wouldn't have shown any obvious signs; she didn't when these happened during the test. When her teachers said they thought she was daydreaming, she was probably having a silent epileptic seizure.'

'What can we do about it?' asked Susan, obviously concerned.

'There are some medicines that can be very effective in

controlling this sort of seizure,' I said, reassuringly. 'We should start treatment cautiously, building up the dose until we have a level that is in the right range. We'll try a slow-release version of a medicine called carbamazepine, so that we can get cover for a whole day, and see whether it helps.'

Nowadays we might use a more modern treatment. The main problem with carbamazepine is that about one in ten patients have an allergic reaction to it. Luckily, Geraldine didn't have this reaction.

It took us several weeks to make sure that Geraldine was well controlled on her medicine. At school, the change was dramatic. She went from being near the bottom of the class to the top two or three. It was clear that the temporal lobe seizures she had been having were the reason for her struggles.

The family kept in touch. Geraldine obtained excellent GCSE and A-level results, went to university and eventually found a career in the banking industry.

PAULINE

Complaints about daydreaming at school crop up not infrequently in paediatric clinics. Pauline Brown was another such case. Her referral letter mentioned her prowess at sports and listed her academic achievements. Lately, though, she hadn't been doing quite so well since turning thirteen and her teachers were at a loss to explain it.

Her mother, Jenny Brown, was also puzzled. She worked in a local pharmacy and had been reading up about her daughter's problems.

'Pauline has always been such a high achiever. She loves her school and always throws herself into everything. Until recently, she has been very successful with her schoolwork and her sports. But nowadays, although she still cares about her work, she doesn't seem to be able concentrate. She daydreams at home too, but we've put that down to adolescence. I think it's more than that.'

The history had been taken by one of my SHOs, who had also carried out a clinical examination. When she had finished, I came into her clinic room to review her findings and go over the case.

'What conclusions have you come to?' I asked.

'I'm not sure what the problem is,' said Dr Jean Murdoch, cautiously. 'It may be just a lack of concentration, as one sometimes can see in young people of this age. I suppose it might have a neurological basis, but I couldn't find any clinical signs to suggest that she had a neurological problem. Syncopal (fainting) attacks could be underlying it, but her blood pressure and cardiovascular system are normal.'

'Thank you,' I replied. 'What do you think is going wrong?' I asked Pauline.

'Well,' she said, 'How would I know? That's why I'm seeing you, isn't it?' Rather a typical teenager's response!

'All I want is your perspective,' I said. 'What do you feel is going wrong, if anything? After all, only you can tell me that.'

'It's not very clear to me either,' she responded, somewhat mollified. 'I seem to lose focus for a moment in class and then I think I've missed a point. I'm not sure why though.'

I decided to take a risk. I picked up a sheet of A5 writing paper from the desk and sat next to her. I held the sheet of paper so that it dangled in front of her nose and mouth. She gave me an odd look.

'I would like you to blow at this sheet of paper while I count up to 100,' I asked. 'I will count for you.'

'What for?' Pauline asked.

'It's just a little test,' I said. 'It may not show me anything, but I think it's worth a try.'

'All right,' she replied.

We started. 'One, two, three,' I counted, as Pauline blew the paper, so that it swung away from her face each time. 'Fifty-one, fifty-two ...' Pauline stopped. I had been watching her closely. Her eyelids flickered for a few seconds during the pause. Then she started blowing the paper again.

'It's all right, you can stop now.'

'I thought you wanted me to count to 100,' said Pauline, clearly a little confused.

'You don't need to now,' I said. 'We've got the answer we needed. Did you see what happened?' I asked Dr Murdoch.

'She stopped before you asked her to.'

'Anything else?'

'No.'

'How about you, Mrs Brown?'

'Her eyes went funny for a bit.'

'Exactly,' I said. 'The point of the over-breathing exercise is to get Pauline to blow off some of the carbon dioxide in her blood. This will push the Ph (acidity) of her blood up into the alkaline range. In young people with petit mal episodes, this change can provoke what's known as an absence and that's exactly what happened to Pauline when her breath count reached fifty-two. That's actually quite early in the test. Usually I find it more often take until the mid-seventies.'

Mrs Brown looked anxious.

'There's no need to be very worried at this stage,' I said. 'Petit mal seizures can develop in young girls as they go through puberty. We can treat it with some medicine and, in a year or two, she is may grow out of it, though not certainly. Some young people go on with it for longer.'

Mrs Brown looked dubious. 'It sounds pretty serious to me.'

'It depends upon a couple of things,' I said. 'We'll arrange for some tests, including an EEG, which looks at the electrical activity in Pauline's brain. It's completely pain-free,' I reassured Pauline. 'They will just stick some wires to your scalp and you can sleep for a while, because it can take up to 30 minutes to get enough measurements.'

I turned back to Mrs Brown. 'Pauline is a little older than the children we see with what we call childhood absence epilepsy; she is more in the age group that have juvenile absence epilepsy. Quite a few of these young people have other sorts of seizures as well, but there's no evidence of that in Pauline's case. The EEG will help us to sort that out. From the story and the clinical signs, I think she belongs in a small group who just have these minor absences and who only need treatment for two or three years. Time will tell.'

I discussed the next steps with Pauline and her mother and they left the clinic.

'Wasn't that a bit risky, getting her to over-breathe like that?' asked Dr Murdoch.

'Yes,' I said, 'but it was a calculated one. Now we know what we're dealing with.'

Pauline turned out to have episodes more typical of childhood absence epilepsy, Her absences were completed eliminated by treatment with ethosuximide. Her progress at school resumed its previous high standard. After three years on treatment, it was tailed off and she had no further episodes (that I know of!).

PETER

The importance of carrying out a full clinical examination is secondary only to listening to the story from the parents. Fourteen-year-old Peter was a case in point. Peter's parents, Simon and Clarissa Simmons, were well-to-do and intelligent. Simon was 'something in the city' and clearly well-off. Clarissa was on local committees and did lots of 'good works'. They had three children, of whom Peter, who was now fourteen, was the youngest. His older brother and sister, Anna and Gregory, had done very well at school, but Peter, although he was progressing fairly well, had not been able to match their progress. Simon and Clarissa were certain there was something wrong with him.

Things hadn't been right from the moment he was born. Peter had suffered from intrapartum asphyxia; in other words, he had been short of oxygen during his birth. He had needed quite a long period of resuscitation, after which he had been transferred to the Special Care Baby Unit. During his first thirty-six hours, he had experienced several generalized convulsions of a tonic/

clonic type – jerking of all his four limbs. None had lasted very long and he was treated with a medicine to control them.

However, after this he did well, thriving at home, and was able to stop his seizure treatment after about six months. His early development was normal and his local paediatrician discharged him from his clinic when he was three.

By the time Peter went to school, Clarissa and Simon felt that something wasn't right. Peter had rather an extravert personality and tended to say exactly what he thought. Tact didn't seem to be something that they could teach him. This led to some awkward moments both amongst the family and later at school.

They sought expert help from various specialists. Peter, over the years, had been seen by paediatricians, child psychiatrists, a clinical psychologist and two professors of paediatric neurology. Their joint conclusions were that Peter was at the mild end of the autistic spectrum and that he was suffering from Asperger Syndrome, a condition in which people are socially less aware, tend to speak loudly, often about one thing obsessively and have less social empathy. Listening to the story and observing Peter in the clinic, this seemed an entirely reasonable conclusion.

However, the Simmons' preoccupation was why this was the case. They wanted to know whether his behaviour could be linked to his problems at birth. Although none of the opinions they had sought had thought that it was, they were unconvinced. They were certain that there must be a link.

I tended to agree with them, although the other eminent professional opinions didn't. After all, as I have often said,

Mother Is Always Right!

I asked Peter whether it would be all right if I were to examine him.

'Not again!' he protested. I could understand his reluctance.

'Well,' I replied, 'I promise I will just carry out a few clinical tests, just to see what I can find.'

'All right,' he conceded.

First of all, I did a stressed walking test, just as I had with Geraldine, asking Peter to walk on the outsides of his feet. He made a fuss about doing it, but eventually tried to. Just as Geraldine had done, his right elbow flexed a little and his hand turned down and inwards as he walked like this. 'Aha,' I thought. I asked him to carry out the piano-playing exercise with alternate hands. Again, just as Geraldine had done, he was unable to 'play' with his left hand without moving the fingers on his right hands. I examined his tendon reflexes. They seemed a little more brisk on the right than the left and his plantar responses were equivocal.

'Did he ever have any imaging tests carried out on his brain?' I asked Clarissa.

'Yes,' jumped in Peter. 'The last professor I saw last year did one where I had to lie in a tunnel for half an hour; it was an MRI. It was very boring.'

Clarissa interrupted. 'He said it was normal, but we asked for some copies of the pictures. We've brought them with us.'

'Please may I see them?'

Simon delved into the capacious briefcase he had brought and pulled out a folder. I took them from him and put them up on the clinic X-ray boxes. They were really interesting.

'Have you looked at them before?' I asked.

'Yes,' said Mrs Simmons, 'but they don't mean much to us.'

'Come and look at them.' They got up and came over.

'I agree that there aren't any obvious *lesions*, but there is one quite striking abnormality. Here are Peter's two cerebral hemispheres: the two halves of his brain, and the MRI scan has produced what one could call a 'cut' in the vertical plane through them in the middle. Next to this I've put another 'cut', made in a virtual horizontal plane. If you compare the two pictures, it is quite clear that Peter's right cerebral hemisphere is significantly smaller that his left, and that the ventricle on that side, this dark space in the middle, is larger on the right than on the left. Taken together with the physical signs I have found with his walking and his finger-wiggling, I am sure that, firstly, these changes are the result of an injury to his brain at birth and, secondly, they are the reason behind his problems with learning and behaviour.'

The Simmons were beaming with relief. 'We were *sure* that was why,' she said. 'Thank you.'

'I'm afraid that, other than giving Peter the sort of psychological and learning support that he is getting already, I don't have anything more to offer. It would be worth carrying out an EEG. I know he has already had one, but my colleague in that department here is really good and I would value his opinion.'

'Certainly' said Simon Simmons. Peter wasn't so keen. When the result came back, it didn't show any sign of epilepsy.

One must always believe what parents tell you. I did wonder whether the Simmons might take legal action about his care at birth, but not a bit of it. All they wanted was to know why Peter had his problems and, having laid that concern to rest, they were happy.

2.

Breathlessness, Sometimes Noisy

OCTAVIA

Sometimes the logic behind a referral doesn't seem to make much sense. Octavia's parent, Jill and Barney Freeman, lived in Devon. Octavia was five months old and had been born in the local maternity hospital. Mrs Freeman's pregnancy, her first, had been uncomplicated and her daughter was a good weight at birth. All seemed well and breastfeeding was fine. The family went home happily.

After that, things began to go wrong. Octavia became difficult to feed, often stopping shortly after starting. With persistence, her mother got through her feeds, though they took a long time. A local breastfeeding adviser came to help, but Octavia didn't seem to be growing very well. Her GP couldn't find anything the matter, so arranged for a local paediatric consultation. There, Octavia was seen by a paediatric registrar who, after discussing the case with her consultant, decided that it was a feeding problem. Another nurse expert in infant feeding was brought in, but Octavia made no progress.

Jill Freeman's mother lived in Cobham. Apparently, she had

heard that I might be a useful second opinion, so arrangements were made for Octavia to be referred to me by her grandmother's GP. All very convoluted, I thought. The family came up to stay with granny in Cobham and Octavia duly arrived in my clinic with her parents.

Barney was a farmer. He wore a three-piece tweed suit and carried a tweed trilby. He spoke with a pronounced Devonshire burr and was sweating heavily. It was a very hot day. Jill was comfortably built and was wearing a more practical floral dress.

Often the best course of action is to find out what the parents think, so, having taken a background history, I started out.

'Tell me about Octavia's feeding,' I began.

'Well,' said her mother, 'She is very slow. I put her to the breast and she latches on quite well, but, after a minute or two, off she comes! Then I wait a bit and can get her back on again and then she does it once more. Eventually, we get a reasonable feed into her, but it can take up to an hour to get through it. We've checked the amount she is getting each day and it should be enough, but she isn't putting on any weight. I simply don't know what to try next. They keep telling me that it's a feeding problem, but can't tell me why she has one.'

There are a few odd facts about feeding volumes. If a baby isn't gaining weight and seems to be getting enough to eat, sometimes it may be that the team haven\t realised that you have to give a baby enough milk to grow *according to the weight they ought to be*, not the weight they actually are. In Octavia's case, it turned out that she was getting enough breast milk.

As we explored her problem, I noticed that Octavia's

breathing was rather faster than I thought it should be. 'Does she ever seem to you to be breathless?' I asked.

'Yes, sometimes,' Jill replied.

'When?'

'Well, sometimes when I am feeding her,' she said. 'Also on one or two other occasions, but I thought she was just getting over-excited.'

I felt it was time to have a proper look at Octavia. We undressed her on her mother's knee. To me, the cause of her problem was immediately obvious.

Octavia at rest was breathing a little faster than normal and she was a little pale, although not anaemic. There was obvious intercostal recession. This is a sign that the lungs are stiffer than normal. There can be a number of causes for this, but I could also see visible pulsation of the heart against the chest wall. The abnormality was clearly cardiac. I listened to Octavia's heart. She was old enough to want to keep trying to pick the stethoscope off her chest. I have a little trick that prevents this. While I examined her, I blew gently upon her right hand. Octavia looked at her hand and moved it about, not understanding why it felt odd to her. She completely ignored the stethoscope on her chest. I could hear a loud pansystolic heart murmur. Together with some other signs, I had the diagnosis and her pallor was the consequence of her heart problem.

'Octavia's problem is the result of having too large a volume of blood passing through her lungs. This is having two effects. Firstly, it makes her breathless, and, secondly, her heart is working extra hard to pump this additional blood, so is consuming more energy and, therefore, more of the calories in her milk. There is less available for her to grow, as a result.'

'What's the reason for this?' asked Barney Freeman.

'I think that there is a big hole between the two main pumping chambers of the heart; what we call a ventricular septal defect, or VSD. As a result, too much blood goes through the lungs, because the resistance to flow there is less than around the rest of the body. She will need a procedure to close this hole, which may be possible to carry out through a special catheter, or possibly a heart operation, but both are standard techniques with very good outcomes. Once the hole is closed, Octavia will thrive, I promise.'

Both parents were visibly both relieved and anxious.

'How soon can this be done?'

'Quite soon,' I said, reassuringly I hoped. 'I will ask one of my colleagues in the children's heart surgery department to see her, today if possible. They will need to carry out some imaging investigations and other tests. Then they will help you decide what to do next.'

Octavia's VSD was closed surgically, as it was rather large. She thrived after that and had no more problems, so far as I know.

One should not be too critical about Octavia's initial consultations in Devon. Heart murmurs can be difficult to hear in babies, especially early on. This is because the resistance to blood flow through the lungs is higher immediately after birth and falls over the succeeding days and weeks. As a result, the heart murmur of a VSD may be very soft initially, but gets louder later on as the lung blood flow resistance falls. Her heart murmur was loud for me, but may not have been so obvious at the time of her previous consultations.

ANABEL

Anabel Sweet was a delightful little girl of seven. She brought several dolls into my clinic, accompanied by her two-year-old sister. Between the two, a complicated game of families evolved, involving their pushchair, a table, two small chairs and some cloth nappies.

The letter from her family doctor simply said that she didn't like walking and complained a lot when the family went for a walk.

This didn't seem too unusual to me. Everyone knows the syndrome of children who moan and complain when walking, without there being anything wrong with them. I wondered what had driven Mr and Mrs Sweet to ask for help. Patrick Sweet was a small man with a luxuriant black beard. Daphne was taller than he and wore a business suit. She worked part-time as an accountant, while Patrick was a floor manager for ITV.

'Well,' Mrs Sweet began. 'It's hard to explain, really. We live right next to Richmond Park, which is a lovely place to take the children. Plenty of space to run around and lots of things to see and do. Anabel plays in the garden happily, but whenever we go to the park, after a while, all she wants to do is to sit down for a bit. She says her legs are tired, but my friends say that some of their children do this too, so it isn't very uncommon. After a while she will get up and play more, or walk home, or whatever. It's just that it happens all the time and it seems to be a bit more of a problem, as she gets older.'

'Is she breathless at all?' I asked.

'No, not at all. In fact, she ran a short race at the school sports day recently, no more than 50 yards, which she won. She was less breathless afterwards than the others, I thought. I did look specially, because of her complaining so much.'

'Does she ever complain of pain in her legs when she is just sitting or lying; in other words, when she isn't walking or running?'

'Not that I can remember.'

'Has she complained anywhere apart from when you go to the park?'

'Yes, as a matter of fact. Several times when we've been on holiday, or visiting her grandparents, if we go on a longish walk she will complain. It seems to be related to taking more exercise than average, although we don't take them on really long walks, because her sister Lucy is a little too young for that yet.'

This still seemed not much to get very worried about. I checked her height and weight measurements, which were done by the clinic nurse before Anabel came in. They were within the normal range for her age.

Time to find out what Anabel had to say. She was very pleased to talk to me.

'Yes, I'm not very good at running about in the park. Daddy says just get on with it, but Mummy lets me have a little rest. Then I'm all right.'

'What is it that makes you stop?' I asked.

'My legs start hurting.'

'Whereabouts?'

She pointed to her calves, then rubbed the backs of her thighs. 'There.'

'Is it there all the time while you are playing?'

'No, I don't have it to begin with, then it comes on and hurts more and more until I stop for a bit. Then is goes away slowly and I am fine again.'

Now we were getting somewhere. This sounded more specific and I was beginning to have an inkling.

'Please may I have a look at you?' I asked her.

'Oh, yes,' she agreed, 'Lucy and I like playing doctors and nurses!'

Anabel's examination was mostly entirely normal. However, there was a slight suggestion that the left ventricle of her heart was minimally enlarged. Also, the closure of the aortic valve seemed a bit louder than normal to me. I examined her pulses. Her brachial pulses, in her arms, were normal. I tried to find her femoral pulses, in the groin. It took me a while to find them, so I compared them with her brachial pulses. They were definitely weaker in the legs but, more significantly, the pulses in her legs were delayed too far in time behind the arm pulses.

'Well,' I said, 'I know Anabel is having quite bad pain in her legs when she runs about or walks for a long time. I think she probably has a very good reason for it. I think the blood supply to her legs, while fine most of the time, isn't quite good enough to cope when she makes her leg muscles do a lot of work for a longer time. As the muscles work harder, they need more blood to bring them more oxygen. Because Anabel's blood vessels can't quite manage to do this, her muscles complain and cause pain. We call this pain ischaemic and her condition is called intermittent claudication'

'Why can't her blood get to her muscles enough?' asked Mrs Sweet.

I pulled over a sheet of paper and began to draw a diagram. 'The main blood vessel supplying the body from the heart is called the aorta. After a baby is born, a small blood vessel, called the ductus arteriosus that allows blood to bypass the lungs before birth, closes off as it isn't needed any more. Sometimes, the little muscle fibres that close it off are also present in the aorta and, when they contract, they cause a narrowing of the aorta which can sometimes be quite marked. This condition is called coarctation of the aorta. If it is bad enough, it is usually picked up at birth. If it is milder, then sometimes it is picked up later, or never at all! I think this is what Anabel has. She will need to see my colleagues in paediatric cardiology and have some imaging tests, but it's something they can easily put right.'

'Will she need an operation?'

'Probably, although, if it is possible, occasionally they can pass a special catheter though it and stretch the narrow part. They will give you the best advice.'

Anabel's coarctation was surgically corrected and she had no more pain.

GERALD

Although the seminal paper on the use of ultrasound scanning in pregnancy was published by Ian Donald's Glasgow team in 1959, it wasn't until the mid-to-late 1980s that devices were built that sufficiently sensitive to detect abnormalities of the fetal heart. Consequently, the identification of babies with heart defects depended largely upon the observations of parents and the clinical skills of paediatricians. Some unfortunate babies slipped through this net and Gerald was one.

Gerald was an eight-year-old boy of mixed race, his father being Caucasian and his mother Chinese. He was referred to me in the early 1980s by his family doctor in Essex, because he was breathless at rest.

When he walked into the clinic with his mother and younger brother, he was a rather overweight child who was a little breathless, but smiling broadly. This was typical of Gerald; he was always cheerful and uncomplaining. He turned out to be highly intelligent.

The most obvious thing about him was that he was cyanosed – blue, in other words. My immediate thought was that Gerald had a variety of cardiac abnormality know at cyanotic congenital heart disease.

I began to unravel his story.

'My pregnancy was normal.' said Mrs Gentle, his mother. She was a beautiful woman of Chinese parentage. 'Gerald was fine at birth and did well in his first few weeks. Then he was a bit slow with his feeds, from about six months of age, but not so bad that I was worried. Everything seemed to be fine until about eighteen months ago. I noticed that he was more breathless than his friends when they played together, but being Gerald, he never complained about it. Anyway, it gradually became worse and I took him to our doctor, who couldn't find anything wrong and told me not to worry. When we went back for a third time, he referred Gerald to our local hospital. He was examined by one of the paediatric team, who again said there wasn't anything wrong with him and sent him home. They did carry out a chest X-ray, which they said was normal. As Gerald was just as bad, I asked for a second opinion, so our doctor asked you to see him.'

I took the rest of Gerald's history. Apart from his school reports, which were all highly laudatory, there was nothing particularly significant.

When I examined him, the clinical signs were clear; he was cyanosed and breathless at rest. The tips of his fingers showed 'clubbing'; they were slightly bulbous, his fingernail beds were blue and his nails curved both from side to side and from front to back. This effect is seen when the haemoglobin in the bloodstream has had a low oxygen content for a while.

Clinically, his heart was enlarged and I thought that this involved the right side of his heart. However, in his case it didn't seem that there was much intercostal recession: in other words, there wasn't an unusually high blood flow though his lungs. His second heart sound was particularly loud and I thought that was produced by his pulmonary valve closing. This is the valve between the right ventricle and the pulmonary artery that supplies the lungs. There was also a heart murmur during heart contraction, a systolic murmur, which was prolonged, but not especially loud.

This picture, together with some other clinical signs, suggested to me that Gerald had most probably been born with a large ventricular septal defect, a VSD like Octavia, but this hadn't been picked up at birth. The result of this was that his lungs had been subjected to an abnormally high blood flow since a few weeks or months after birth. As I have pointed out in Octavia's case, the resistance to the flow of blood through the lungs falls steadily after birth, so the murmur of a VSD may be almost absent at birth, but gets louder as the resistance falls and the blood flow there increases. That's why VSD murmurs can be easily missed.

The problem with this pattern is that, over time, the high pulmonary blood flow can lead to a change in the blood vessels in the lung and they close down progressively, reducing the blood flow. Eventually, they can close down to the point where the resistance to the blood flow through the lungs is higher than the resistance to blood flow around the rest of the body. When this happens, instead of blood flowing through the VSD so more blood goes around the lungs, flow reverses and more blood goes around the body and less around the lungs. The blood coming back to the body has had much of its oxygen used up, desaturated as doctors call it. The patient becomes permanently cyanosed, or 'blue'. This is what had happened to Gerald and it was bad news.

I sat down with Gerald and his mother and told them what I had found.

Chunhua Gentle was remarkably calm about the situation.

'I knew something was not right,' she affirmed. 'But I wasn't sure what. What should we do now?'

'I will get my paediatric cardiology colleagues to see Gerald. They will have to do some tests. Don't worry,' I said to Gerald, 'Apart from a blood test, the other ones aren't at all painful.'

'I'm not,' Gerald said boldly. 'I think I'll find it very interesting.' He smiled; so typical of him.

They left the clinic, relieved that something would be done.

Gerald's investigations showed that he was not in a good way. He did indeed have a large VSD with a reversed flow across the defect. The blood pressure in his lungs was too high for him to have his VSD closed. It was necessary to try to get his high pulmonary blood pressure down and the resistance to blood flow through his lungs reduced before any corrective surgery could be undertaken.

Although Gerald was seen regularly by paediatric cardiology, he came to see me also, at his and his mother's request. There was little I could do, but they appeared to value my opinion on what was being done to help Gerald.

His medical treatment continued for several years, but we were never able to bring his pulmonary pressure down sufficiently. His heart condition became more severe and, when he was twelve, a request was put in for a heart transplant. In those days, heart transplants for children were uncommon and obtaining tissue matches difficult. It was especially hard in Gerald's case, because of his mixed-race heritage.

We were never able to source a heart for him and he passed away at the age of thirteen. His mother, undaunted, started a charity to raise money for the support of children who needed heart transplants.

If Gerald had presented today, more could have been done to help him, as there have been major advances in the management of these conditions.

The death of children as opposed to newborn babies, is rare in paediatric practice. Gerald was a wonderful boy and his passing still makes me profoundly sad.

SALLY

Children often present with problems with their breathing and we classify them in particular ways. A common type that makes mothers very anxious is stridor. This is a loud noise while the child breathes in. In small children it is usually caused by a virus and is called croup. Sometimes epiglottitis is cause by a bacterium called Haemophilus influenzae and that's a serious problem. This inflammation of the epiglottis, which overhangs the entrance to the trachea at the back of the throat, makes it swell, so that it partially blocks the airway and, on breathing in, the obstruction is worse; hence the stridor. Normally, when you swallow, it folds over the top of the tracheal entrance, to prevent you inhaling food or drink.

Sally Weston was brought to our Children's A&E with stridor. She was nine months old and her mother had gone to pick her up after an afternoon sleep to find her making this loud noise when she breathed. Panicking, she scooped her up and brought her in. Sally was obviously anxious and breathing quickly.

The paediatric team found that she didn't have a fever, so

assumed that it was croup. They gave her a single dose of a steroid, called dexamethasone, and admitted her for observation. I saw her on the ward next morning, when she was still stridulous. However, the noise was a bit odd. It sounded to me too musical to be proper stridor. In addition, Sally was smiling up at me, obvious not in the least distressed.

There was a latex teething giraffe in the cot. I picked it up.

'It's her favourite,' said Amanda Weston, her mother. 'She chews on it a lot, though.' It was certainly well-used.

I bent closely over Sally. She smiled again.

'Could I have a pair of fine forceps, please?' I asked. The staff nurse looked puzzled, but trotted off to find some.

'What do you want those for?' asked Dr Wilson, my registrar. I didn't answer him. The nurse returned with the forceps. I bent over Sally again and applied them gently.

Magically, the stridor disappeared. I confess that, sometimes, I like a bit of theatre.

'What did you do?' cried Amanda Wilson. The team looked startled.

I held up the forceps. I was gripping a small silvery disc with them.

'I thought the noise didn't sound quite natural and, when I leant over, I could see something bright in Sally's right nostril. It's the squeaker from her giraffe! She must have accidental removed it and it got stuck up her nose.'

I told the A&E team about it, because I thought perhaps they hadn't looked at her carefully enough. It was the easiest cure for 'croup' I've ever employed.

WILLARD

Peanuts are the classic object inhaled by toddlers. One such, two-year-old Willard, was admitted to a ward where I was the Senior Registrar.

The peanut was successfully removed by the chest surgeons and, in due course, I wrote his discharge letter.

I dictated it onto a tape as usual and later came to sign it. The first line read:

'Willard had been discharged from the children's ward, having successfully had a *penis* removed from his right main bronchus.'

Our secretary was slightly embarrassed.

ERIC

Eric was another toddler admitted with breathing problems. His mother, Iris Evans, had gone to get him up in the morning and found him with noisy breathing. Iris was a comfortable, blowsy lady with a strong Irish accent. She picked him up and patted him on the back, but that didn't help. As he seemed to be more distressed, she brought him straight to the hospital. Eric had been born to her later in life.

I was in the Children's A&E when they turned up. Eric was a chubby little boy who looked a little anxious. His breathing was certainly odd: he had a noise on breathing in, stridor, but also one on breathing out. We'd normally call that a wheeze, but it sounded a bit different.

'He was fine when I put him down last night,' said Iris. 'He's a very good sleeper and last night he was just the same. I didn't hear anything in the night and I only noticed the breathing when I went to pick him up in the morning.'

'He hadn't vomited during the night?' I asked.

'There was a small posset on his babygro, but nothing out of the ordinary.' she said. 'I've changed it,' she added, defensively.

I examined him. His chest was showing less movement on the left than on the right. On listening to him, the breath sounds on that side were diminished.

'I think he may have inhaled some of his puke,' I said. 'We'll get a chest X-ray done, because it sounds as though he's blocked off a part of his lung with it. If so, we can ask the children's chest surgeons to put a tube down into his airway and remove it. That should do the trick.'

Mrs Evans looked worried. 'Does that mean surgery?' she asked.

'Not exactly,' I said, trying to be reassuring. 'They will give him an anaesthetic and suck it out. There shouldn't be any actual surgery needed.'

She was relieved.

Eric's X-ray showed partial collapse of his left lung, mostly involving the upper lobe. That fitted, because he'd been lying on his back in his cot.

Next day, the surgical team took him to theatre and carried out a bronchoscopy, where they put a tube in his airway. Sure enough, his bronchi contained material that was blocking air from getting in.

The thoracic surgeon, James, rang me.

'It's very odd,' he said. 'I don't think it's come from his

stomach, it's not food. It's a sort of white, fibrous, crumbly material. Anyway, it's out now and he's breathing is fine.'

I returned to the ward to speak to Iris Evans.

'Was there anything else in the cot when you went to get Eric up yesterday?'

'No, not a thing.' She paused. 'No, I tell a lie. There was some white stuff on his cot and on him a bit. I cleaned it off.'

'Where did that come from?'

'The ceiling. Some of it fell down in the night. I've a feller coming round this afternoon to fix it.'

'Good,' I said. 'That's what we found in Eric's chest.'

'Well I never!' she exclaimed.

AUGUSTUS

I first met Augustus when he was about five years old. His family doctor said that he'd had lots of chest infections, since he was about six months old. They had all got better with either conservative treatment – a wait and see policy – or with antibiotics. However, his chest was always noisy when the doctor listened to it and now he was bringing up sputum which was sometimes greenish or yellowish.

This didn't sound at all good. Children rarely bring up sputum unless they have a significant chest problem and the colour of his sputum suggested that it was infected.

His mother, Victoria Chastaine, was a charming and sensible mum.

'I've got four children,' she began. 'They're all very healthy save Augustus. He seems to get everything that's going. He's not growing as well as his brothers and sister, and his chest has begun to be quite noisy too.'

'Aw, Mum!' protested Augustus. As I got to know him, I learned he was very bright and didn't like any suggestion that he was different from anyone else. He hated making a fuss, which may partly account for him presenting rather later than I would have expected.

I took the rest of his history, which was normal. He got lots of chesty infections, but he also suffered from sinusitis.

'Dr Meads says it goes with his chestiness,' said Victoria.

'Please may I have a look at you?'

'All right.'

Augustus took off his shirt and sat on the couch. He was rather skinny and his ribs were prominent. I noticed that he had a slight wheeze and a little recession. This is when the spaces between the ribs get sucked in slightly when one breathes in. I noticed something else. My eyes widened in surprise.

'Doctors have listened to chest before, haven't they?'

'Sometimes,' said Victoria. 'Not always.'

'Which part do they listen to?'

'Always at the back.'

That accounts for it, I thought.

I could see the beating of Augustus' heart on his chest wall. That's quite normal in thinner patients, to be able to see the apex beat. What was wrong here was that it was visible on the *right* side, not, as is normal, on the left.

I examined his chest. Yes, his heart was on the right and not the left. He had dextrocardia.

I continued the examination. I was fairly sure his liver was primarily on the left and not the right; the wrong way round too.

His chest was very noisy, with lots of rhonchi and a few crepitations, signs that there were lots of secretions present and possibly mild pneumonia.

'You have something we call Kartagener Syndrome,' I told Augustus. 'The main problem is this. Your airways are lined with lots of tiny hairs, called cilia, that sweep the mucus that protects them from dust and bugs up into the back of your throat, where you swallow them. In your condition they don't work properly, so the mucus accumulates, makes you cough it up all the time and makes you more likely to get chest infections. The same problem is causing your sinusitis.'

'Can you help him?' asked Victoria.

'Yes, we can,' I said. 'It's not the only thing I've found, though,' I said. 'Something that goes with Kartagener Syndrome is what we call situs inversus. Augustus' heart is on the right and not the left and his liver is on the left and not the right. It probably applies to all his organs that predominate on one side or the other. This doesn't matter at all to Augustus, they work just fine, but we need to know it when we examine things, or we'll look in the wrong place!'

We all laughed. But Kartagener Syndrome is a serious condition and usually leads to lung damage.

Augustus began a lifelong relationship with our physiotherapists, learning how to get rid of his secretions and, with the help of antibiotics, to keep his chest free of infection. He managed fairly well and I saw him regularly until he left my care and went to the adult respiratory medicine team.

I was at a conference once in Barcelona when some cases of Kartagener Syndrome were presented. Afterwards, an older doctor stood up to ask a question. However, he pronounced it as Kartagener Syndrome, with the emphasis on the third syllable, not Kartagener Syndrome with the emphasis on the second syllable, as had the presenter. He foolishly tried to correct the questioner. The questioner replied, gently, 'I am Dr Kartagener.' He had been the first to describe the condition.

ANTHONY

Anthony was the father of a little girl, Petula, whom I met in my clinic. Petula had eczema, which we dealt with satisfactorily over a period of about six months.

It was Anthony's story that was so interesting. As he sat down, he said that his experiences in British hospitals hadn't been ideal. Out came his fascinating medical history.

He was born in London and had mild respiratory problems at birth. Investigations at the time had shown that he had congenital emphysema of the upper lobe of his right lung. In this condition, after birth, the affected lobe of the lung expands rapidly, compressing the rest of the lung on that side. As the abnormal lobe doesn't function, the baby is surviving on one lung.

The classical treatment is to remove the abnormal lobe, but, in Anthony's case, he was only mildly distressed, so they decided to wait and see.

As Anthony thrived, it was decided to leave well alone. He

had a happy and healthy childhood and was able to join in sports with his friends, perhaps becoming breathless a little more easily, but with no real distress. He went to university and qualified as an engineer.

When he was twenty-five, his company posted him to California, where he lived for fifteen years, acquiring an American wife and three children.

In his first year there, he broke his leg while skiing and was taken to hospital. As part of his admission routine, a chest X-ray was taken, which revealed his congenital lobar emphysema. A chest surgeon came to see him.

'No problem,' he said. 'I can take that out for you.'

Anthony wasn't sure this would be a good idea after so long, but the surgeon was very confident. I would have been more cautious, because one might expect the major part of the lung, having been compressed for twenty-five years from babyhood, would be so small as to be non-functional. Anyway, partly because his company was paying his medical costs, Anthony agreed.

The surgery went ahead. Afterwards, Anthony was fine. When his chest X-ray was repeated they found, to Anthony's surprise and relief, the rest of his lung had expanded to full his right chest cavity and, what is more, it had grown with him. His lung function was significantly improved as well.

Anthony brought his X-rays to one of Petula's follow-up clinics. The right lung was a little more clear than the left, but the difference from normal was minor.

I found this, from a medical point of view, quite extraordinary.

3.

Mostly Mewling and Puking

HENRIETTA

Infants and toddlers under two are delightful, but two problems often drive some parents to despair. Some of them scream whatever parents do to try to calm them down, while other puke all the time, creating lots of extra washing, as if there wasn't enough to begin with! Most of these young children have nothing seriously the matter with them, but one or two may have causes that require treatment. As a paediatrician, the trick is to be able to identify the healthy ones and reassure their parents, while not missing those who may be suffering from a serious illness.

Henrietta both screamed and puked. This one-year-old toddler arrived in my clinic, brought by her mother, Sheila Almond, who had a harassed look, and accompanied by one of her siblings, Paul, aged four. The other, Julia, who was six, was at school.

'She used to puke a little when she was a newborn baby,' said Sheila, 'But this was normal, I thought, like Julia and Paul. But they settled down by about six months and stopped when I began them on mixed feeding. Henrietta's just got worse. First of all, she started to vomit more and more, volume I mean, and after I started to wean her, it didn't stop at all.'

'When does she vomit?'

'A little while after she feeds. Sometimes after I put her down to sleep.'

'What does she bring up?'

'Only what she's eaten.'

'There's no blood or yellowish-green bile in it?'

'No.'

'When does she scream?'

'All the time!'

'Well, she is being very good now.'

'She fell asleep on the way here and has only just woken up. You wait!'

'Is there any pattern to her screaming?' I asked.

'Not really, but it seems to happen more when I'm cleaning her up.'

'How does she sleep at night?'

'Actually, quite well for the last six months, thank goodness. She used to cry a lot at night, but now she sleeps through. At least we all get some rest now.'

All this suggested that there wasn't anything serious behind her screaming other than habit. I would reserve judgement.

I looked at her growth pattern, comparing her measurements in the baby follow-up clinic and her measurements on that day. Her growth was fine, although there was a slight suggestion of slowing over the last month or so.

I took a full history of the pregnancy and birth, all of which were normal, and there wasn't anything in the family history of concern.

'Have you tried thickening her feeds?' I asked.

'Not really,' Mrs Almond replied. 'But it hasn't got any better now she is on more solid food.'

I examined Henrietta carefully, without finding anything amiss. I turned to Sheila Almond.

'The most likely cause is what we call gastro-oesophageal reflux, which is quite common in babies and almost always gets better on its own eventually. I think, for the moment, we should do two investigations, provided you agree. First of all, I think a plain chest X-ray would be a good idea, just to make sure everything is where it should be. Then, I can arrange for her to have a special test where we see what happens to some fluids we'll give her that shows up on X-ray. It's chocolate-flavoured, so Henrietta will probably lap it up. While we are waiting for those test results, I can give you a sort of gel that you add to her drinks, which will make them a bit less sloppy in her tummy, so that they don't come up so easily.'

'Why has she got this gastro-oesophageal reflux?'

'That's an interesting question. The reason lies partly in the anatomy of the upper part of a baby's stomach. The oesophagus runs into the stomach at a slight angle and there is a ring of what's known as smooth muscle around the lower end. In babies, there is less oesophagus below the diaphragm than when they are older. Also, newborn babies' stomachs don't make much, if any, acid. This is because the production of stomach acid is stimulated by a hormone called gastrin and babies produce very little of that. Gastrin also causes the ring of muscle to contract, helping to stop food coming back up after eating. Good sense, really, because the hormone that makes stomach acid helps to prevent heartburn!'

'You can see from this that the muscle ring can't work at birth, so babies have to rely on something called the "pinchcock mechanism". This depends upon the acuteness of the angle at which the oesophagus runs into the stomach. As this varies quite a lot in babies, some babies puke a lot, where it doesn't work very well, and others hardly at all, where it does. Then, as gastrin production gets high enough, the ring of muscle begins to contract after a meal and the puking and/or vomiting stops.'

'It may be that Henrietta has a hiatus hernia, of the kind we see in infants sometimes. If there is very little of the oesophagus below the diaphragm, then the pinchcock mechanism doesn't work at all and it takes much longer for the effect of gastrin to be enough to close off the stomach. The special tests will show us.'

'Let's wait and see if this helps and, perhaps, her screaming will gradually go away.'

The reason for carrying out a chest X-ray first was to make sure there wasn't any important abnormality, such as a diaphragmatic hernia, present. In this condition, there's a hole in the diaphragm and, if there had been one on the left side, it might have explained the vomiting. But there wasn't. The chocolate barium swallow showed that Henrietta had quite marked gastro-oesophageal reflux and that there wasn't much oesophagus below the diaphragm.

Luckily, the thickening agent help to reduce her vomiting, although it went on for another three or four months. Once it had stopped, it didn't return. The screaming stopped too. All was well that ended without any more puke.

ABDUL

Sometimes, simple clinical routines can save a lot of confusion.

Abdul was born at our hospital, following a normal pregnancy. His mother was healthy after the birth, but developed a low-grade fever, so stayed in for a day or two. She started to breastfeed, but Abdul proved a bit difficult to feed, so artificial feeds were started. He didn't do any better on these, continuously regurgitating the milk that he was offered.

After four days, he was becoming dehydrated and so he was transferred to one of my wards. Here, he was seen by my SHO and the Registrar, Dr Heeney. They agreed that Abdul was a little dry, so started him on intravenous fluids that evening.

I came in early the next morning, and, before my regular ward round, popped in to look at Abdul, because no one was sure what the problem was.

He was still mildly dehydrated and he also had a slightly anxious look about him. You might think that a five-day-old baby can't have an anxious look, but I would disagree with you. That's probably because I have seen a lot of babies.

I carried out a thorough physical examination, but otherwise he was entirely normal. I asked the nurse for a nasogastric tube and some litmus paper.

'What for?' she asked.

'You'll see in a minute,' I replied.

She came back with an unsuitable 8 French gauge tube and the litmus.

'That's too small,' I said. 'Please may I have a 12 or 14 gauge tube?'

'He's only a small baby,' she said. 'Dr Heeney managed with an 8 gauge one.'

'Aha,' I said, mysteriously. 'That may explain things.'

She came back with a suitable tube. I attempted to pass it through Abdul's nose into his stomach. After a few centimetres, it wouldn't go any further. I tried two or three more times, then stopped.

'Okay,' I said, 'Let's get the team together.'

We met in Sister's office.

'He's got oesophageal atresia,' I announced. This happens when the oesophagus doesn't develop properly and ends high in the chest. It explained Abdul's anxious look. He must have been wondering when someone was going to feed him properly.

'He can't have,' objected Dr Heeney. 'When I looked at him, I passed a tube into his stomach quite easily.'

'How do you know?' I asked.

'It went all the way,' he insisted.

'Did you suck up an aspirate and check it for acidity.'

'No, because a newborn's stomach doesn't make much acid.'

You will remember, in Henrietta's case, I mentioned this, but at birth there *is* quite a lot of stomach acid, stimulated by maternal gastrin.

'The stomach pH will be acid when tested by litmus paper,'

not wanting to waste time pointing this out. 'You used an 8 French gauge nasogastric tube, I think.'

'Yes,' he replied.

'Well, that's the problem,' I said. 'If you employ too thin a tube, it can coil itself up when you try to pass it. You won't know whether it has reached the stomach unless you test it. I used a 14 French gauge tube and it stuck in the upper thoracic position. He's got oesophageal atresia. Let's get the paediatric surgeons involved.'

Abdul was rapidly sent off into the care of the paediatric surgeons who specialise in correcting these abnormalities. During foetal development, the upper end of the oesophagus and the lower end migrate slowly towards each other. When they meet, they fuse and a hollow tube develops, running from the pharynx (throat) down into the stomach. Sometimes they sort of miss each other and the baby is born with an oesophagus that ends in a blind tube. The ease of a surgical repair depends upon how much of the lower end on the oesophagus is present below.

In Abdul's case, there was enough for the surgeon to join the two ends together, just about.

The other problem associated with this is the presence of a fistula (a connecting tube) between the upper end of the oesophagus and the trachea, known as a tracheo-oesophageal fistula, or TOF. Abdul did have one, but, fortunately, it was quite small, so very little of the feeds he had been given seemed to have gone through it into his lungs. The fistula was tied off and the remnants removed.

Abdul needed quite a lot of expert post-operative care with

his feeding, but everything went very well and he grew into a happy and healthy little boy.

Had we been more alert in the immediate post-natal period, we might have picked this problem up much sooner. It's a routine procedure to pass a nasogastric tube in a baby who presents with this kind of feeding difficulty. Of course, you must use a big enough tube.

MADELEINE

Madeleine was a delightful five-year-old girl who lived in Kent. She was referred because she had been suffering from recurrent unexplained episodes of vomiting since she had been a baby. Her family doctor's letter described these bouts as not having any especial significance to them, but they seemed to occur, nowadays, every two weeks or so.

Sometime after a meal, she would complain about a pain in her tummy.

'I always know when she's going to vomit,' said her mother, Emily Sturridge. 'She always points to a place just to the left of her belly button. Then we pick up her bowl – we always have one to hand – and wait until it's over.' Emily seemed to have a strong grasp of her daughter's problem. She was a primary school teacher.

'What does she bring up?'

'Usually it's partially digested food. What she has had, if it's soon after a meal. If it's later on, it's a bit mushier. We try to give her food that's not too lumpy, as she can manage that without vomiting better.'

'It is ever greenish-yellow in colour?'

'Not that I've ever seen.'

'Does she have a noisy tummy?'

'Not really.'

Other than a tendency to minor constipation, Madeleine was quite well and her growth was within normal limits. On my clinical examination, I could find nothing wrong.

Quite a lot had been done at her local hospital. She had been a regular visitor there and eventually was reviewed on several occasions by her local paediatricians. They had arranged for various investigations, which included both a barium swallow and a barium meal. In these two tests, you persuade the child to swallow a liquid barium mixture, usually flavoured with chocolate, and take some X-ray pictures. The swallow looks at the mechanism of swallowing and the meal looks at what happens after food reaches the stomach. Both these tests had been reported as being normal.

'Did you bring the X-rays with you?'

'Yes.' Emily Sturridge gave them to me. I put them up, one by one, on the X-ray box and we looked at them together.

I was intrigued.

'This is the stomach here,' I said. 'Then, if you look carefully, you can see the next part of the bowel, which is called the duodenum. But it doesn't look quite right to me. This is the first part of the duodenum and, as you can see, it's quite full. Then, here's the next part, which is less well defined. If you look carefully,' and I pointed this out, 'There is a faint darker line running across the end of the first part. Can you see it?'

Mrs Sturridge wasn't convinced. 'I can't make that out,' she said. 'What would it mean, anyway?'

'I suspect that Madeleine has a partial duodenal web,' I replied. 'When the bowel is developing, this happens by various solid parts joining together and turning in tubes. Sometimes, the development of the cavity doesn't quite go all the way and a child can be left with a membrane closing off the bowel, with just a small hole in it. In Madeleine's case, it means that well digested runny food can get through, but not really solid food.'

'Why did they report it as normal?'

'Well, it is very difficult to see and it is a bit easier for me because, having seen you and Madeleine, it was one of the things I was looking for,' I said. 'Also, you have general radiologist at your local hospital and they wouldn't be so used to looking at tests from small children as my specialist colleagues here. We need to have better pictures than this and a video of the barium going through that area would be helpful. I will have a chat with my colleague in paediatric radiology.'

'What can we do about it?'

'If it proves to be the problem, Madeleine would need a small operation to remove the web, but it would be a complete cure.'

'Oh goody,' said Madeleine, 'I'm fed up of my vomiting!'

Madeleine, with her mother, went off to book her test. When we got the result, it confirmed that she had a partial duodenal web. This was removed surgically and she made a complete recovery.

GRAHAM

Graham was a boy of twelve who had been affected by intermittent episodes of abdominal pain and vomiting for several years. He lived near High Wycombe and his family had lived in the area for many years.

We're kind of an institution in the village," said Eamon Mason, his father. "There have been Masons there for over five hundred years"

"And so have my folks," Mrs Mason chimed in. "We know that the Sadlers, my family, have been around at least as long, from the gravestones in the churchyard."

"Does that mean that you are distant cousins?" I asked, alert to the possibility of a genetic abnormality.

"Not that we know of," replied Olive Mason. "I suppose, going back, it's quite likely, but not in the recent past. We met at the village school, but we think we must have known each other before that, though we can't quite remember."

Interesting, I thought, because Eamon and Olive Mason looked very much like brother and sister!

Graham's GP had written me a long referral letter. It seemed that the Masons had been bringing Graham to his surgery ever since he was about a year old, because of his episodes of tummy-ache and vomiting. They weren't all that frequent; he had been known to go for up to six to nine months without any, but they always started up again. Sometimes it was just tummy ache, at other times Graham would vomit for a few hours, then it all settled down. As he could find nothing wrong, at first, he put it down to bouts of food poisoning, or of viral gastro-enteritis, but their repeated nature made this seem less likely.

He asked for the local paediatrician to have a look at him, for the first time when he was six. Nothing abnormal was found, but Graham was referred to him twice more over three years. They had carried out lots of investigations, including stool cultures and imaging studies of his bowel, but everything was found to be normal. Finally, a decision was made to ask for the help of a child psychiatrist.

This specialist agreed that there seemed to be an emotional fragility about Graham and had begun sessions of CBT, cognitive behavioural therapy, the previous year. These are so-called 'talking therapies' with one-to-one sessions with the therapist. There had been eight sessions so far, up until just before I met Graham. In that time, he had experienced two more of his bouts of pain and vomiting. The Masons had asked for a second opinion, hence his appearance in my clinic.

I thought that it wasn't at all likely that the problem was psychological. After all, they had started when he was a year old and been continuing, on and off, for eleven years. No, there was something organic going on.

"Do you know when you're going to have one of your vomiting bouts," I asked Graham.

"Not until I get my tummy pains," he replied. "I don't always have the pains either, sometimes I just feel a bit sick and start vomiting."

"When you have the pain, where is it exactly?"

Graham pointed to the middle of his abdomen.

"What does it feel like," I asked. "Is a steady pain, or does it come and go?"

"Yes, it seems to come and go for a while. It stops after I've been sick."

"What comes up?"

"Usually a sort of mishmash of food," he said, screwing up his face. "But sometimes nothing very much, just some greenish fluid."

"Does your tummy sound noisy sometimes?"

"Yes, it does. Funny that. I can be lying in bed and I think it is talking to me, it makes all sorts of gurgles."

"Do you have episodes of diarrhoea or constipation?" I asked.

"Only sometimes," Graham replied "And they're not when I have my bouts of vomiting."

Mrs Mason chipped in "We wondered about that, but his bowels are regular most of the time and, if he does have a problem, it's rare and nothing to do with this problem."

All this suggested that Graham had intermittent intestinal obstruction.

"Did you bring any of his X-rays with you?"

"We don't have them. They're all at the hospital," said Olive Mason.

"All right," I said. "As this has been going on so long and Graham has had so many tests, I think the best thing is for us not to do any today."

Graham looked very pleased.

"I think that the problem is almost certainly caused by what is actually quite a minor abnormality in your bowel." I said to him. 'It's difficult to spot on X-ray, but I think I may be able to tell, if I can have a look at the ones you've already had. I will ask your local hospital's radiology department to send them to me and I will take them to our weekly X-ray meeting.'

'What do you think is wrong, exactly?' asked Eamon Mason.

'When the intestine is developing in the unborn baby, it goes through various stages. At a late one, it rotates around its attachment to the back of the abdomen, in order to end up in the normal place, with the appendix on the right side and the large bowel all around the outside of the cavity. Sometimes this doesn't happen, or only happens partially. This is called a malrotation of the intestine, although, more correctly, it's a *failure* of the bowel to rotate in the usual way."

"Why does this cause Graham's vomiting?" asked Olive.

"If malrotation is present, the bowel isn't tied down in the right place. Sometimes it twists around itself and causes a blockage, Then, after a while, it untwists itself and the obstruction clears. You can see that this fits quite well with Graham's symptoms and the fact that they get better of their own accord."

"If that's the problem, then Graham would need a small operation," I said.

Graham didn't look very pleased about this.

"It's very simple, the surgeon sort of ties down the bowel, so it can't move around."

"Would he put it back in the proper place?" asked Eamon.

"Definitely not! If you do that, sooner or later it frees itself and the problem recurs. All he needs to do is to make sure that the bowel can't twist and that's quite a simple job."

The Mason left, looking hopeful. A couple of weeks later, I had Graham's X-rays from his local hospital and took them to our X-ray meeting. I had already had a quick look at them.

The plain X-ray of his abdomen was suggestive, but the Barium study showed that he had malrotation. A few weeks later, Graham had his operation and his problem was solved.

TALULAH

Talulah was a baby of nine months of age, admitted while I was SHO at a children's hospital. She had been admitted because she was failing to thrive and her mother, Lily Thorne, thought she wasn't able to swallow properly.

She came in from the consultant's clinic, with instructions for a number of investigations. I took a full history and arranged for the tests. When we got the results, the cause was clear. There was a large mass at the base - the top end - of her heart. This mass encircled her major blood vessels, her trachea and her oesophagus. We didn't know what it was, although it seemed unlikely that it had an infectious origin, as her investigations didn't show any signs of infection.

We had a meeting with Talulah's parents. My consultant explained the findings.

"What can we do next?" asked Mrs Thorne.

"We'll need to ask our surgical colleague to see her. I hope they'll be able to get a sample of the tissue in this lump, so we can find out what it is."

"What do you think it is?" Lily asked.

"We don't know yet, that's why we need the biopsy. Let's get that done before we speculate."

We had, on the staff, one of the greatest paediatric cardiothoracic surgeons in the world. He agreed to take her theatre, carry out the biopsy and try to assess what might be feasible from a surgical point of view, if an attempt at removing this mass was needed. He wasn't hopeful.

We waited for the biopsy result. It wasn't good news. First of all, the mass was a malignant neuro-endocrine tumour. In adults, these are very rare and often secrete hormones, but in children, where they are extremely rare, they usually don't do this. Secondly, our surgical colleague said that the position of the tumour and its likely invasion of local organs made surgery impossible.

We pondered on what to do next, before speaking to the parents again. We felt we needed to offer them something.

"Is there any cytotoxic (cell-killing) drug we could try?" I asked, innocently.

"These cancers are very resistant to the drugs we have. It's unlikely," responded our expert, the oncologist.

"What about some that act in unpredictable ways?" I persisted. "I know there have been some remarkable successes."

"We could try Vincristine," he suggested. This is a cytotoxic drug derived from the periwinkle that is used to induce remissions in lymphoblastic leukaemia. "We could give it a go."

We met the parents and passed on the bad news first. They were very distressed.

"We think it's worth having a go with a cancer drug, Vincristine," said my boss. "We don't know whether it'll be helpful, but we think it's worth a try."

"Please," they said.

"We worked out an appropriate regime for Talulah and

started treatment. For a week or so, Felicity remained in her obstructed state. Then she seemed to improve a bit.

"Do you want another chest X-ray?" I asked my boss and the oncologist.

"No, let's wait a bit longer. We can see that she seems to be better and we need to give it a bit longer. We can keep the number of X-rays down at the same time."

We waited for a month. Talulah was much better, Indeed, her parents thought she was back to normal.

We repeated the chest X-ray. The mass had vanished. We never found any sign of it after that.

Talulah went home completely cured. We could never say whether it was the result of treatment with Vincristine, or whether the tumour regressed on its own. What did it matter, so long as she was cured?

LLOYD AND LAWRENCE

Lloyd and Lawrence were nine-month-old non-identical twin boys. Their mother, Imogen Weeks, was a single parent who had given up work when her twins were born and was planning to go back to her job as a receptionist, once her boys were settled and she could find suitable childcare. She had no close family living nearby. However, although Lawrence was growing well and thriving, Lloyd was not. They were both being seen regularly by the community paediatric team, so they were being monitored frequently and the difference in growth patterns recorded.

Imogen started breastfeeding both twins, but found that

she couldn't manage it, so they moved over to artificial feeds. Lloyd's growth began to fall off around this time, at about a month of age and before the introduction of a weaning diet. This made some conditions like cœliac disease less likely, but didn't exclude a sensitivity to cow's milk protein or some genetic abnormality.

The community paediatricians arranged for a series of investigations, all of which came back normal. Lloyd didn't seem to have any symptoms; he didn't behave differently to Lawrence in any way. Imogen reported that he fed well, opened his bowels normally and had as many wet nappies as his brother. It seemed that there was no obvious reason for Lloyd's failure to thrive. The community doctor discussed it with me and agreed that a period of observation in hospital might be helpful. At the same time, we could look for more obscure metabolic and hormonal reasons for his growth failure.

Ms Weeks was very unhappy with this suggestion. I suggested that they could all come in, mother, Lloyd and Lawrence. This was more acceptable and was arranged.

Imogen was determined to provide all the baby care herself. This was perfectly fine with us, but we found it a bit odd that she was so insistent. In due course, the family arrived and were given a large room to themselves.

Having all the family together proved to be very helpful. We arranged for the additional investigations and instituted a programme of careful monitoring of feeds. Immediately, we ran into a problem. Imogen wanted peace and quiet to feed the twins and wouldn't let any of the staff sit with her during feeding times. We thought this was rather peculiar and decided to weigh both babies several times during the day before and after feeds, to determine how much feed each was getting.

This proved to be rather tricky. Imogen contrived to make it difficult, finding all sorts of reasons why this couldn't be done. Eventually, we resorted to weighing the boys when she was out of the room, when she went to the restaurant for her meals, for example. We also noticed that Lloyd had significantly fewer soiled nappies than his brother and didn't wet them as often either.

A pattern was emerging. I suspected that Imogen was not feeding Lloyd much at all, but giving plenty of feed to Lawrence. This is a pattern that has been described before, called 'scapegoating', a form of Munchausen by Proxy, in which an illness is manufactured by a carer, usually a mother, who seeks repeated medical advice for an artificially induced illness.

Proving it in this situation would be very difficult. I had several gentle and sensitive discussions with Imogen.

'We are worried about Lloyd, as you are. Perhaps it would be good for you to have a rest every now and then and let the nurses feed them sometimes.'

'No, I'm going to do it myself. Everyone seems to think that I can't manage them on my own and I'm going to show them that I can!'

'I understand that, however, it is very tiring doing it on your own, especially when one of them isn't well. It would be good for you to have a break.'

'I don't need a break. I can cope.'

We had several more conversations along these lines.

We discussed the situation amongst the team. Everyone was convinced that Lloyd was, basically, a healthy boy and that Mum was the cause of his problem. But Imogen refused to be budged. A confrontation became inevitable, as Lloyd's poor growth was becoming critical.

'I think it's important that you leave the children with us for a bit.'

'Absolutely not!'

'Well, if you won't agree to that, I will have to ask for us to have the care of your babies for the moment.'

'You'd better not!'

I sought an emergency care order, which was granted.

'Imogen, I am afraid that we can only allow you to be with Lloyd and Lawrence under the supervision of one of the nursing staff and you won't be allowed to be in with them during feeding times.'

My announcement was greeted by screaming, threats and imprecations. However, I had legal control of the boys and we started to get on with feeding them ourselves. Imogen would be outside their cubicle when they were fed, always angry that we wouldn't let her in.

Slowly, Lloyd began to grow at a more normal rate, then more quickly and, over a fairly short space of time, he almost caught Lawrence up. The only thing that had changed was that he was getting enough food to allow him to grow. This, of course, was only solving the first part of the problem. What could we do to make it possible for the boys to go home?

Having obtained an emergency care order, we had to arrange

for a review with social services. As Munchausen by Proxy is a form of child abuse, representatives of the police, from their child abuse team, also attended. The first meeting needed to be held within two weeks of the granting of the emergency care order, ideally as soon as possible. This was too soon for us to be able to show that Lloyd was now thriving, but it was agreed to allow us more time.

By the time of the next meeting, his improvement was striking. Everyone agreed with our diagnosis. What next?

Munchausen by Proxy is a parental illness. We needed to persuade Imogen to have a psychiatric assessment and to have treatment, usually some sort of 'talking therapy'. This was something I couldn't do because, understandably, I had become the object of Imogen's hatred. 'It's all your fault!' Our wonderful ward sister had managed to strike up a fair relationship with her, so she eventually was able to obtain Imogen's agreement. After all, it was the best way for her to have her children back.

In the meantime, we developed a plan of supervision to be put in place when the boys were judged to be allowed to go home safely. All of this took some time and their admission had lasted over eight weeks by the time we were in a position to let them go.

For the same reasons, I did not arrange for them to see me in a follow-up clinic. Fortunately, there was a community paediatric clinic close to their home, so they were seen there on a regular basis and social services kept a close eye on them at home, dropping in unannounced sometimes.

Why, you may wonder, would Imogen treat her children

so differently? No one can say for certain, although one can speculate. First of all, she was a vulnerable single mother, living with twins as her first children, which is extremely stressful. Secondly, it turned out that she had few, if any, friends. Thirdly, she had rather an abrasive personality, tending to push people away. Underneath all that, she was probably desperate for attention; exactly why she sought it in this unusual way, I have no idea, but it certainly worked.

I am glad to say that the two boys both made really good progress after this.

GEORGINA

Georgina Ellis was a nine-year-old girl from East Sussex. Her GP asked me to see her, because she was not gaining weight at a normal rate and she was rather pale. She came to my clinic with both her parents and her six-year-old brother Sebastian. Paula and Peregrine Prentice were a professional couple. Paula ran an interior design business and Peregrine was a stockbroker.

Georgina's family doctor said that the Prentices were a family that were alert to healthy living. In other words, they were likely to sign up to the latest dietary fad. Like all parents, they wanted to ensure that their children led as healthy lives as they could make them. Plenty of physical activities meant that both were involved in sporting clubs outside their private schools: mini-rugby for Sebastian and netball for Georgina. Of course, they also played sports at school as well. Parents such as these lead quite stressful lives, juggling work and supporting all these extra children's activities. The referral letter was a very full and helpful one.

I knew that this would be a difficult consultation. I would need to be extra careful not to tread on any parental prejudices. I began cautiously, talking around the problem.

'Gosh,' I started, 'Your children lead busy lives! It must make a lot of work for you.'

'Well,' said Paula, who was the dominant character, 'It's what one does, isn't it? Children are *so* important, aren't they? And one only gets one chance to get it right.'

'You are so right,' I said, sycophantically. 'There isn't a reliable guide to what is the right thing to do, though there's lots of advice around.'

'I know,' she said eagerly. 'I try to keep abreast of what's out there and pick up what seems to be best.'

More discussion followed before I thought it was time to focus on Georgina.

'Tell me about Georgina's problem,' I asked, being careful not to specify.

'I'm not sure there is much to worry about, really,' Paula said. 'Yes, she hasn't gained weight so fast lately, but there are other girls skinnier than her. She can be picky at mealtimes but show me a child who isn't.'

'Apart from that, you don't have any concerns about her health?' I asked.

'No, not really.'

I looked at Georgina again. She was a pale blonde wisp of a girl who was happily reading a book she'd brought with her. Sebastian was reading a picture book.

'Your doctor thought she looked a bit pale.'

'She always looks like that,' Paula said, defensively. 'After all, blonde girls usually have that sort of look.'

Georgina, to me, seemed extremely pale, so much so that she was clearly anaemic.

'What sort of diet does she eat?' I asked.

'Well, we have been concerned about all the additives there are in foods and the propensity for young people to develop allergies, so, after lots of debate, we became vegan a couple of years ago.'

'So, how has that affected your children?'

'Oh, they are all very keen on the idea. They like that we're protecting animals and not eating them and they seem to have taken to the alternatives very well.'

'Is Georgina eating the same as the rest of you?'

'Yes, though she has been a bit more picky than Sebastian, as I mentioned.'

'What would she eat on an average day?'

'She has breakfast, though usually that means some orange juice and a cereal biscuit, because she doesn't like the muesli we eat.'

'Does she eat a school lunch?'

'Yes, but she takes a packed lunch that I make myself, full of lots of the right foods.'

I looked at Georgina. She blushed. 'Do you eat it all, Georgina?' I asked.

'Some of it,' she admitted.

'What happens to most of it?'

'I give it to my friends. They like it.'

'Don't you?'

'Not very much,' she admitted.

I turned back to Paula. 'Does she eat a good supper when she gets home?'

'Well, not as good as I would have liked. We try to have lots of vegetables, but Georgina won't eat them. She eats some carbohydrate, like potato or pasta or rice.'

'What about protein?'

'She isn't that keen on the alternatives we have, like nuts and so on.'

'How does she manage at the weekend?'

'Well, she'll often say she isn't hungry. I try to tempt her, but she's very reluctant.'

I went on to try to take a full dietary history. Georgina was not actually eating very much at all. In particular, her diet was low in protein and extremely low in iron.

I had a thorough look at her. She was markedly anaemic and rather thin, her weight being well below what one would have expected for her height. Her tongue was rather smooth, another indication of iron deficiency.

'I think Georgina is short of quite a number of elements that she needs in her diet. Her intake of protein is on the low side, but, more importantly, she is very anaemic. Of course, there can be lots of reasons for this, but I suspect it's just that she isn't getting enough iron in her diet. This will have lots of other effects, for example on her behaviour and on her learning.'

'But she is doing quite well at school!'

'Good, but perhaps she could do even better. Also, it may be that, if her iron status improves, she may eat more healthily. We see that effect quite often.'

'What next?' said Peregrine Prentice, looking more interested.

'We'll need to carry out some blood tests first. I think we should give her some iron supplements now, because it is just possible that may be all we need to do. One thing you need to be aware of; vegan diets are fine for most people, but not ideal for children. That's because there are some nutrients that one can only get from animal sources, whatever the populists may say. One of these are what we call polyunsaturated long chain fatty acids. The shorter ones are available from plant sources, but human metabolism can only add a fixed number of extra chains to lengthen them. Really long chain ones are very important for brain growth and, to make these, shorter ones have to go through more than one animal. Babies get four steps, from grass, to cows, to mother and then their own process. Children can have three steps on a mixed diet, but only one step on a vegan diet. Cow's milk is a good way to give the right mixture to them.'

'But I'm worried about them becoming allergic to cow's milk!'

'Do you have a history of allergy to cow's milk?'

'Well, no,' said Paula.

'Then give it to them. I'm sure they'll be fine.'

Paula looked dubious, but agreed to give it a try and to risk them having eggs as well.

When we had Georgina's test results, she had very little iron on board and her haemoglobin level was 4 g/dl, a third of what it ought to have been. Fortunately, the Prentices both made sure that Georgina took her iron medicine and modified the children's diet sufficiently that she put on weight and was no longer anaemic. Interestingly, her dietary fads disappeared, and she went to the top of the class.

Everyone knows about appendicitis, but not many people realise that it can present in some different and confusing ways in children.

SIMON

Simon was an active and happy little boy, until, one day, when out with his mother at the local playground, he complained of pain in his tummy. Mrs Reid thought that he'd simply overstrained himself and, with words of encouragement, took him home. She offered him some tea, but he wasn't interested. This being very unusual for him, she became more concerned, so she took him to see their family doctor.

Dr Peters had a look at him. Simon's pain was on the lower left side of his tummy. Although it wasn't the intermittent, colicky sort of pain he would have expected, he thought Simon was constipated and sent him home, asking his mother to telephone him if he didn't settle down. A couple of hours later, Simon vomited, although he hadn't eaten or drunk very much. Mrs Reid thought he had a slight fever. She rang the GP, but got the answering service and, after listening to his symptoms, they recommended that she take him to A&E.

They arrived at my hospital and were seen by the doctors in the Children's A&E Department. They noted that he was still constipated and had a slight fever. They thought he was tender in his left iliac fossa – the part to the left and below his belly button. They weren't certain what was going on, so they admitted him to the ward. Observations were made through the night, every hour.

I saw him early the next morning. He was still complaining of pain in the same place and his low-grade temperature had continued. A blood count suggested that he had some sort of infection, probably bacterial, with raised markers of inflammation and a raised neutrophil count.

Mrs Reid was looking anxious. 'What's wrong with him?' she asked.

'Something we can sort out very quickly,' I said, reassuringly. 'Just let me go through this with the team.'

I turned to Dr Smithers, an SHO. 'You can see that he is still slightly feverish and still tender in the left iliac fossa. Did you notice anything about his tenderness?'

'Yes, she said. 'There was some rebound tenderness, suggesting peritoneal irritation.'

You find this sign when the peritoneum, which lines the abdomen, is inflamed.

'What should we do next?'

'Send off some blood cultures and start him on antibiotics.'

'Sorry, no, I meant what else should we do clinically?'

Dr Smithers wasn't certain. I asked Dr Shaw, the Registrar.

'I know it's not so easy in children, but I think we need to carry out a rectal examination.'

'Spot on. Why?'

'In case he has a left-sided appendix, with appendicitis.'

'Full marks. Let's do it.'

I explained to Mrs Reid that, in a few people, their appendices are on the left side, instead of the right. This can lead to appendicitis being easily missed, or mistaken for something else.

Simon's rectal examination revealed the signs of left-sided appendicitis. We called our paediatric surgical team, who took him to the operating theatre. They found his inflamed appendix, which had not ruptured, and removed it. He also had malrotation of his bowel. Simon made the usual speedy recovery that children often do and went home happy and well.

SAUL

Saul was a six-year-old boy who had been taken ill at school after lunch. He complained of pain in his tummy, vomited and developed diarrhoea, all in the space of a couple of hours. The school was concerned that he had gastroenteritis as a result of his school dinner, so they began a check on the food preparation that day. In the meantime, his mother collected him from school and took him to our Children's A&E Department.

There, our doctors found central abdominal pain and tenderness and a fever of 39 degrees centigrade. His vomiting and diarrhoea were continuing. The provisional diagnosis was that he had gastroenteritis due to a bacterial cause, possibly due to an organism known as campylobacter. They carried out a series of blood tests, sent of a stool culture, put up an intravenous infusion so that food and drink could be stopped while he was vomiting and admitted him to my ward. All very thorough.

When I saw him later on, he wasn't really any better. I examined him. His abdominal tenderness was more severe than I would have expected. In addition, it seemed to me that he was particularly tender in his right iliac fossa and that, like Simon, he had some rebound tenderness. My team weren't very impressed.

'The rebound isn't very marked; it could just be his inflamed bowel.'

'It's just because his right colon is sore.'

'Yes, those are all reasonable explanations,' I agreed, 'But what must we exclude?'

'Well,' said Dr Raynes, the SHO, 'Could he have a retro-caecal appendix?'

'Exactly what I am worried about,' I said. 'Let's arrange an ultrasound of that area and get the paediatric surgeons to look at him afterwards.'

The caecum is a small sac at the beginning of the colon and close to the appendix. Our further investigations showed that Saul had retrocaecal appendicitis. This was irritating his colon and causing his diarrhoea.

Saul had successful removal of his appendix, after which all was well.

JULIA

One Saturday morning, on my ward round, I saw Julia Stirling. She was an eight-year-old girl who had been admitted, complaining of central abdominal pain. This had been going on for several days and her mother, Veronica Stirling, had taken her to their GP about it twice.

On the first visit, Dr Flew noted that she had a slight, but significant fever and examined her. Seeing that one eardrum was a little inflamed, she had made a diagnosis of otitis media (an infection of the inner ear) and prescribed a course of amoxicillin, an antibiotic. This is not an entirely conventional thing to do, because most ear infections of this type, without a high fever, are caused by viruses, so an antibiotic won't make much difference. But it wasn't an unreasonable thing to do and probably kept Mrs Stirling happier than simply telling her to wait and see.

The fever lasted a couple of days, but Julia's tummy ache got worse. It was still around her belly button, but she found it hard to say whether it was a constant pain, or whether it came and went. This latter is what we call 'colicky pain' and tends to be associated with bowel problems.

Her GP had another look at her and couldn't find anything wrong. As Mrs Stirling was rather anxious, she sent her to our Children's A&E Department. Our team had a thorough look at her and also found nothing wrong, apart from the pain. She was still on the antibiotic. Their provisional diagnosis was mesenteric adenitis.

When children develop an infection, this stimulates their immune system, which in children can react quite vigorously. The bowel hangs from a membrane called the mesentery with has many lymph nodes in it. These enlarge in response to the infection and stretch the mesentery, which has lots of pain fibres in it. It is one of the assumptions often made in paediatrics that this is why children often complain of abdominal pain when they have an infection. The evidence that this is actually what happens is thin, though I find it a convincing idea.

The doctors in Children's A&E arranged several investigations and admitted her for observation on the children's ward. This might sound rather a drastic step for a child who only had a tummy ache, but, as there was no definite diagnosis, we felt it was safer to do this for a day of two. Often the cause becomes clear.

Julia" tests showed a raised neutrophil count and raised ESR and CRP levels, suggesting some sort of infective cause.

I sat on Julia's bed and spoke with her.

'My name's Colin. I've come to see you about your tummy pain.' She looked at me doubtfully.

'Have you still got the pain?' Julia nodded. 'At the moment?' She shook her head. 'Does it come and go?' She nodded again. 'Does it come and go and come back again quickly, almost immediately, or does it come back after a longer time, like five or ten minutes?'.

'Longer,' she said, briefly.

Getting answers to questions like this is difficult in young children, because their concepts of time are a bit hazy. It seemed to me that this wasn't a colicky pain, however.

Further questions showed that she hadn't been eating or drinking a lot and was constipated. Her charts didn't show any fever. I began to examine her; she was a very compliant child, often a sign that a child isn't very well. She had, also, a slightly washed out look.

When I examined her tummy, she was less compliant, but I was slow and gentle. After a while, I was certain that she had significant tenderness in her right iliac fossa. I turned to Mrs Stirling.

'I think Julia has appendicitis,' I said, to her surprise. 'I think her symptoms have been modified by her course of antibiotics.'

'I need to do a rectal examination and to arrange for an ultrasound of her abdomen. I will ask for the surgeons to have a look at her.'

Mrs Stirling wasn't keen on the rectal examination, but I explained why it was important. When I did this, I was sure that there was confirmatory tenderness on the right side. I continued my ward round.

Later that day, I got some feedback. In the ultrasound department, they couldn't find anything wrong in Julia's abdomen. This was odd, but, being at the weekend, the radiologist on call wasn't specialised in examining children and might have missed it. The surgical Senior Registrar on call had a quick look at her and pronounced, 'If this is appendicitis, I'll eat my hat!' Dangerous words, thought I, because he wasn't a paediatric surgeon, hadn't examined the child and had made too many assumptions. I decided to wait.

Julia's pain continued, but was not too dreadful for her. We managed to control it. Monday morning arrived. I telephoned our expert paediatric radiologist and our excellent paediatric surgeon and explained the situation.

Later that morning I had two telephone calls.

'I've had a look at Julia's abdominal ultrasound,' said the radiologist. 'She's got an appendix abscess.'

'Why have you been sitting on this child?' raged the surgeon, crossly. 'I'm taking her to theatre this afternoon.'

I breathed a sigh of relief, but the Senior Registrar in surgery never ate his hat.

ZAK

I made a diagnosis in Zak's case, having never seen him, from 800 miles away. Sitting at my desk, eating a sandwich while doing some paperwork one lunchtime, my telephone rang.

'Hello', I said.

'It's Peter Smith', was the reply. He was a colleague of mine whose specialty was Elderly Care. 'Could I ask you for your advice?'

'Of course. I'm in my office having a sandwich. Why don't you come now?'

'I can't. I'm at Son San Joan Airport, in Palma, Majorca!'

'Oh, that's difficult,' I replied, lamely. 'How can I help?'

'It's my son, Zak. He's six. He started to be unwell last night, he's vomited a couple of times and now he's complaining of tummy ache. I thought he had gastroenteritis, but it doesn't seem quite like that. He's not had any diarrhoea and he has only a slight temperature. What do you think?'

'Have you felt his tummy?'

'Not really.'

'Check to make sure he doesn't have tenderness in his RIF.' That's his right iliac fossa, where the tenderness of appendicitis is usually located. There was a pause.

'Yes, he seems to be a bit tender there.'

'Well, an airport isn't the easiest place to do a rectal

examination. When do you fly home?'

'In about 30 minutes, we're about to get on our plane to Gatwick.'

'Okay, I'll get someone to meet you.'

I got busy on the telephone. Within an hour, I had arranged for an ambulance to meet them off the plane and bring him to our hospital and arranged that our paediatric surgical team would be ready in the operating theatre about two hours after touchdown.

Zak arrived an hour after they landed. We confirmed the diagnosis, did the necessary test and his inflamed appendix was removed two hours after he landed. I never actually saw him, because I was busy at another appointment.

FELICITY

Some parents become very focussed on their children's bowel habits. Twenty-month-old Felicity was one such child. Her GP had written to say that Felicity's parents reported that she opened her bowels four or five times every day, that her motions were very soft, even a bit runny and that they could see undigested food present in them.

There is a perception that the presence of undigested food in a stool must mean that the child in question has some sort of failure to digest food normally and this shows there is a disease present. Actually, it doesn't usually mean anything of the sort, but it causes lots of anxiety.

Mrs and Mrs Foster arrived with Felicity in a pushchair. They seemed to fill most of the space in my clinic room. Both parents must have weighed over 125 kg each, although Mrs Foster was larger than her husband. I looked at Felicity, who filled her pushchair. She was a very large toddler indeed. This was clearly not a case of failure to thrive!

'Hello,' I said. 'How can I help you?' wanting to see how the land lay.

'It's Felicity's bowels. She opens them far too often. Her motions are very runny and I can see some of the food I have given her in them,' said her mother Rachel.

'What is it that you think might be wrong?' I asked, innocently.

'Well, it's obvious,' said David Foster. 'She's not digesting her food properly, so it's running out the other end!'

'I see,' I responded. 'What do you give her to eat each day?'

'When she gets up, she has a rusk with some milk. Then we have breakfast and she'll eat cereal or porridge, followed by eggs, fried or poached, with some baked beans. She'll drink some orange juice and some milk. Mid-morning she'll have juice and some biscuits and she eats a good lunch. Possibly ham, egg and chips, or shepherd's pie, with some veg. Then cake and custard for dessert. She'll have more juice at teatime with a sandwich – I cut the crusts off for her. At dinner time she eats with us and has the same as we do, but I will mash up some of the foods for her. Then some milk before she goes to bed.'

I had been totting up the calories as we went along. Felicity was being given more than double the amount of food that a child of her age would need, at a conservative estimate. The reasons for the family sizes were apparent.

'Please may I have a look at Felicity?'

'Of course.'

There was then rather a struggle to get her out of her pushchair. She was wedged in!

'We've been meaning to get her a bigger one,' said Mrs Foster.

When Felicity's growth was plotted, although she was tall for her age, her weight, in proportion, was far above the appropriate level for her height. At least, in other respects, she was healthy.

'Does she sleep well?' I asked.

'Yes, though she snores quite a lot,' said Mr Foster.

'But we all do,' injected Mrs Foster.

I am sure that both parents had obstructive sleep apnoea and Felicity too, probably.

'Well,' I said, slightly apprehensively. 'It's clear what the problem is here.'

It was important not to be too confrontational at this point.

'There is no need to worry about seeing recognisable food in Felicity's stools. When you see this, it's because food is moving through the bowel so quickly, not all of it gets digested. The next question is why this is happening.'

'Is it serious?' asked Rachel Foster, anxiously.

'Not at all,' I replied. 'You can see that Felicity is much larger than other children of her age.'

'It runs in the family,' said David Foster.

'I can see that. But it isn't good for Felicity to be as large as this, and you can do something about it. You are offering her rather more food than she actually needs, so we need to help you to manage that.'

'But she's always hungry!' said Rachel.

'The more you give a healthy child like Felicity, sometimes the more they'll want. In her case, the amount of food she is eating is the reason it's all rushing though her bowel and coming out the other end with some undigested. We don't need to starve her. We'll get one of our special children's dieticians to work with you. Between you, Felicity will have a diet that is the right amount nutritionally, but won't leave her hungry. Would you be happy with that?'

'Well,' said Rachel Foster, 'If it stops her diarrhoea, that'd be good.'

We made the necessary appointments. I followed up Felicity in my clinic for a few months. Her bowels slowed down and she began to produce a normal stool once or twice a day. Her weight gain slowed and, though she would always be a larger than average child, moved closer towards the correct weight for her height.

Sometimes, the cause of the problem is staring you in the face.

CHARLES

On holiday, being a paediatrician carries the risk of being asked all sorts of medical questions, so, although I'm always willing to offer help, I don't advertise the fact. When our children were pre- and early teenagers, we took them on a series of activity holidays around the Mediterranean. Our first one was on the Turkish coast, near Bodrum.

I was playing volleyball on the beach against some local

Turkish boys, when another guest tapped me on the shoulder.

'Are you the paediatrician?' he asked.

'Well, yes, but how did you know?' I replied, taken aback.

'I didn't,' he said, 'But someone came and asked me if I was one, but I'm an anaesthetist and he said that he'd been told there was one here, so I've been going round trying to find you.'

'How can I help?' I asked, realising there must be a clinical problem somewhere.

'Apparently, there is a nine-month-old baby boy who has been ill for the last day or so and his parents don't know what to do next. They've only been here three days.'

I was aware that a couple had arrived at that time with two children, a baby of nine months, a daughter of five years, plus a nanny. I also knew that they had gone to Ephesus the previous day, leaving the boy with their nanny, because I had seen them leave. We didn't go, because we'd been to Ephesus before. I asked whereabouts they were and set off to find them.

I met the parents, Amanda and Julian Richardson-Smith, near the bar. They were extremely worried about their little boy Charles. When they set off for Ephesus, Charlie was fine. When they returned, he had started to vomit. The vomiting continued, so they sought the advice of a local doctor, who diagnosed viral gastroenteritis, recommending that they maintain him of clear fluids for the moment. However, the sickness continued overnight, accompanied by sparse loose stools. This morning, he had also passed some small bloody stools. Panicking, they had sought me out.

They took me to see Charles, who was on the nanny's lap.

Her name was Victoria. He looked a bit dehydrated.

'Please may I have a look at him?' I asked her. She loosened his clothing.

As he was distressed, I placed the whole of my hand gently on his tummy. In babies, this is a good way to get a general idea of what is going on. I think I must have stiffened a little as I did so, because Amanda reacted.

'What's wrong?' she asked.

'Give me a moment,' I said.

Under my hand I could feel a mass about the size and shape of a large sausage, running across his abdomen at a slight angle. It was firm, without being hard and, from Charles' reaction, slightly tender. I knew immediately that this was an intussusception.

In this condition, the small bowel becomes tucked inside itself, rather like turning a sock partly inside out. The waves of peristalsis that pass along the bowel, to move food along, catch hold of one of the lymph nodes that line the bowel and this acts as a tug, pulling the bowel along behind it, inside the bowel further on. In children between six and eighteen months, small bowel lymph nodes are often rather large and it is thought that this is the reason that the condition occurs at this age.

It's a paediatric emergency. He was a long way from the right help.

'Charlie has got part of his bowel stuck inside another part of his bowel, like a partly inside-out sock. He needs to see a children's surgical team. He may need an operation to pull the bowel out again, although, if we are quick enough, putting a tube into his bottom and blowing air inside can sometimes do the trick.'

The Richardson-Smiths were distraught, as you might imagine.

'What on earth shall we do?' exclaimed Julian.

The manager of the resort was a great help. From him, we established that the nearest suitable hospital was the Children's Hospital at Izmir, 240 kilometres away, just over a three-hour drive. He telephoned them and they said to come at once. The manager offered to drive them there and take his barman, who was a trained nurse. The five of them set off, leaving nanny Victoria with their daughter, Petronella.

Four days passed, during which we all had a good time and hoped that all was going well. Then Amanda and Julian returned on their own, in a taxi. I was a bit worried. However, it was all right, they just wanted to ask my advice. It seemed a long journey to do that, perhaps they could have phoned me, I thought. They told me how Charlie's illness had progressed.

'When we got there, they whisked him away,' said Amanda. 'We weren't allowed to stay with him. They sent us to this nice five-star hotel next door. Soon, they told us that Charlie did have an intussusception and that they had pushed it back with air, as you said they might. They asked us to come round to collect his blood tests and take them to the pathology department a block away. We did that several times. Charlie did very well so, this morning, they said we could take him back. We went to pick him up, but then he puked all over me. "Whoops", they said and took him back, had another quick look at him and said he now needed an operation, as his bowel has some damage. They've taken him to theatre and we got very worried again.'

'From what you've said, it sounds as if they've done all the right things.' I reassured them. 'They have picked this up quickly and, being a baby, he'll probably do very well.'

'Yes, well, we'd rather get him back to England when they let him out,' said Julian.

'Do you have travel insurance?' I asked. This was in the days before such insurance was compulsory.

'Yes.'

'Where do you live?'

'Claygate, in Surrey.'

'Oh, that's very convenient,' I said. 'It's in my hospital's catchment area. We're going home in two days' time. I will make sure there's a bed for him and you can arrange, through your insurer, to fly him home. They will want to know which hospital he's going to.' I gave them the details.

Two days after my return to work, Charles appeared on my ward. Apart from a scar and a small stitch abscess which we drained, he had no more problems.

Two years later, we were on our third multi-activity holiday, this time in Crete. One evening, at dinner, I sat next to a lady who extracted from me that I was a paediatrician.

'Oh,' said she. 'I heard a good story about a paediatrician on one of these holidays.'

She then regaled me with Charlie's story, with embellishments. Apparently, I had operated on Charlie's intussusception on the holiday resort's kitchen table! I didn't enlighten her; it would have spoiled her fun.

4.

Bladders and Related Bits

Bedwetting is a problem that the general paediatrician is asked about quite often, usually a boy between six and eight years old who has never been dry at night. More common in boys, possibly because the urethra, the tube that connects the bladder to the outside, is longer in boys. Sometimes, children don't become dry at night until about six to eight years old, so it's a good idea to wait and see, if the child is younger.

LEWIS

Lewis Peterson was a typical eight-year-old in this category. He'd never been dry at night, but his older sister was dry at three and his five-year-old brother had been dry for a year. His failure to become dry at night stood out a bit and he was, as you might expect, embarrassed about it.

His GP has offered the usual advice, but thought Lewis had reached the age when he needed a buzzer connected to a mesh sheet in his bed that caused an alarm to sound if his wet the bed.

He came with his mother, Ann Peterson. She was a pleasant lady in her late thirties. She wasn't too worried about Lewis' bedwetting.

'His dad has been more impatient with him, not that he has anything much to do with the washing! It's really Lewis who would like to be dry. Then he can go on sleepovers.'

'Oh yes please!' said he.

I took a history and examined him. He was a healthy boy and had no anatomical abnormalities of his external genitalia that I could see. His parents, unlike some, had been patient and tolerant over his problem. Some parents get very stressed and upset, often making the child feel more guilty and tending to poison the relationship between parent and child. Needless to say, this usually makes the situation even worse.

My approach to this problem was always a little unconventional. I always made sure there is no urinary tract infection present and arranged for an ultrasound of the urinary tract, a useful non-invasive test. I always asked the ultrasonographer to check that the child emptied the bladder completely after passing urine, as a residual volume of urine is a potent cause of recurrent urinary tract infections.

I arranged these tests, but I decided to treat Lewis as though his investigations were all normal.

'Lewis, please come and sit on my lap.' The paediatrician of today would not do this, because it would be considered a most inappropriate thing to do. My reason for doing so was that I was going to talk to Lewis about his peeing and, in my experience, embarrassed little boys will look all around the room and shut you out if they sit in a chair, but, once on your lap, they do pay attention to what you are saying.

'Lewis, I'd like you to think about how you feel after you've gone to bed and you're about to drop off to sleep. Can you imagine that?'

A nod.

'Okay, not I'd like you to pretend that you are bursting to go to the toilet to pee, but instead, I'd like you to squeeze off tight down below, to stop yourself from peeing. Can you do that?'

Another nod.

'Now, what I would like you to do is, at home, every night when you are about to drop off to sleep, try pretending again, just like that, then relax, then squeeze tight again and do that six times. Then you can go to sleep. Can you remember to do that?'

A final nod.

'Don't worry, I'll remind him,' said Mrs Peterson. Of course, I knew she would. I gave her a star chart record sheet, so that she and Lewis could note the nights he was dry or wet. If he managed five nights in a row, he would get a gold star.

'I'll see you again in a month and we'll see how you've got on.'

Four weeks later, Lewis came into the clinic with a grin on his face. 'I'm dry,' he announced, obviously pleased with himself. We looked his chart. It was almost all gold stars, as he had only had one wet night since I had seen him, two nights after his first clinic visit.

'That's brilliant,' I said. 'And all your tests are normal too,' I added.

I found that, with this management, eight out of every ten children I saw with bedwetting, providing they had no other problem with their urinary tract, became dry. Very rarely did I need to resort to electrical or other devices.

PAULINE

Pauline Doherty was twelve years old. She lived in Reading and was suffering from several years of recurrent urinary tract infections (UTIs). They were first identified when she was only nine months old, picked up by an alert GP. She gave her a conventional course of treatment which got rid of it, but, a month or two later, back it came. Wise to the possibility of an abnormality of her urinary tract, she requested a paediatric consultation at their local hospital.

She was seen there and all the appropriate investigations were carried out. Her imaging studies showed that she had a condition known as bilateral vesico-ureteric reflux (VUR), quite common in children who have frequent UTIs. When these children empty their bladders, although most of the urine is passed, some goes back up the ureters towards the kidneys, so at the end of micturition (peeing) this urine drops back into the bladder.

Normally, bacteria pass quite easily up the urethra, the tube from the outside to the bladder. Passing urine, so as to completely empty the bladder, is the most important way you protect yourself from UTIs. If there is a residual volume of urine, you can see that it's likely there will be a high risk of lots of UTIs.

The point at which the ureter enters the bladder is the critical one. There is no sphincter. If there were, it would be a ring of smooth muscle that could close off the ureter and prevent urine flowing back up towards the kidney when the bladder contracts. Instead, the ureter enters the bladder wall at an angle.

As a result, when the bladder contracts, the bladder muscle acts to close off the end of the ureter. There is significant variation in the angle at which the ureter passes through the bladder wall and this means that there is consequential variation in the efficiency with which this 'pinch-cock' mechanism works. For this reason, VUR isn't all that uncommon.

Pauline was only fifteen months old at the time the reason for her recurrent UTIs was established. She started on prophylactic antibiotics; these are low dose antibiotics particularly suited to preventing UTIs, often because they are excreted unchanged in the urine. For quite a few years, these did the trick. however, from the age of eight or nine, Pauline began to suffer from occasional UTIs, often with organisms resistant to her usual preventative treatment.

At this point, I was asked to see her.

'It's getting to be a real nuisance,' complained Pauline. 'When it happens, I leak a bit and this is embarrassing at school. My friends know all about it, but they don't really understand.'

'How often do you pee?' I asked.

'Much more often when I have a UTI.'

'Does peeing become uncomfortable?'

'A bit, but I've got used to it. It's a helpful signal.'

'Do you take a long time over peeing?'

'No, I just go more often.'

'How often?'

'Sometimes ten times a day or more.'

'Do you go several times close together?'

'Not usually. There's at least twenty minutes between.'

This was very helpful and I now knew what we might be able to do to help. Pauline had been examined many times and had always been found to be healthy, but I did the routine things. Importantly, her blood pressure was still normal for her age.

She had undergone a series of recent investigations at her local hospital and she had brought a thick folder with all her results in it, including the imaging results.

'May I have a look at those?'

'Of course.' Mrs Doherty handed them over. Pauline was a bright and mature young lady, so Mum had left the consultation to her. Mary Doherty was obviously proud of her daughter's ability to manage the consultation on her own.

Pauline was presently on a new antibiotic, for a short course, to get rid of a new UTI. I looked at her recent imaging studies. Her kidneys remained normal; a relief in view of her long history. She had undergone a recent nuclear imaging investigation, in which one can track urine from the bladder, on peeing, to see whether it is flowing back towards the kidneys. It showed that this was still happening to a significant degree.

'Has anyone suggested that an operation to re-implant your ureters into the bladder could be tried?'

'Yes, but we looked into that and the results are very variable. We didn't think the risk outweighed the possible benefits to Pauline,' said Mr David Doherty, who was, by chance, a statistician.

'I think you are right,' I said. 'Although there are some newer techniques, such as the injection of fillers around the ureteric opening, that are more helpful. However, I think, in the meantime there is something quite simple that you can try. Triple micturition.'

'What's that?' asked Pauline.

'It needs a bit of planning on your part, but it is often very effective. Try to set times aside for your pees every day. You'll need about 15–20 minutes, so clear it with your school. Go to pee as usual, then wait five minutes and go again. Wait another five minutes and go a third time. You must do this all the time, every day. Because you have VUR, waiting five minutes allows the urine that's gone back up towards your kidneys to fall back into the bladder. Each time this will be less, but there will always be some to pass. If we can keep the residual volume of urine in your bladder as low as possible, that will reduce the risk of infection. Of course, you will still need your preventative antibiotic treatment, but this will cut down the risk of a breakthrough infection.'

'I'll give it a go,' said Pauline.

I did review Pauline in my clinic a couple of times. However, after this visit she had no more breakthrough UTIs while she remained a paediatric patient: at least four years. Simple solutions should never be ignored.

A common complaint of the parents of newly born girls is that their external genitalia are too large. Of course, when one looks at them they are quite normal, but they look slightly out of proportion, due to the influence of maternal hormones reaching them in the uterus. Some parents take a bit of convincing.

The circumcision of girls is a completely unacceptable

operation, but that of boys is a more nuanced subject. Some religious practices, such as Islam, require that it is carried out. While working in the Middle East as a visiting professor, every morning newborn boys would be lined up to have their operations carried out, amid a chorus of protesting yells. In Britain, male circumcision is not allowed under the NHS for socio-religious reasons, but only where there is a medical indication, such as phimosis. This is a condition in which the foreskin becomes narrowed and is restricting the boy's ability to pee.

Occasionally, boys would be referred to my clinic because both their parents and the GP considered that phimosis was present.

'I am unable to retract his foreskin properly' would be the complaint. And therein lay the error.

First of all, in baby boys the foreskin isn't capable of full retraction, because it is slightly adherent to the glans penis it covers. Secondly, in older boys, the way to check this out is NOT to try to retract the foreskin at all, but to grip the foreskin gently on either side by the thumb and first finger of each hand and to PULL it outwards. When one does that, in most cases, lo and behold, a wide passage opens out, demonstrating that it is not causing any obstruction to the flow of urine at all. It is also a very good way of demonstrating its adequacy to the parents. It is quite difficult to retract the foreskin anyway, because the trapped of excess foreskin tissue beneath the overlying part makes it harder.

Another common complaint is that of undescended testes. These are usually boys of five years old or more, who have had a recent medical check for some reason. In over 70 per cent of cases, there is nothing wrong.

The best time to check whether the testes have descended into a normal position is at birth. Normally, they migrate into the scrotum before birth and once there, they stay in position. As boys become older, the testes become retractile, so that, in situations of stimulus, like fear, or on examination, the retraction of testes high in the scrotum is quite common. The examining doctor fails to find them, so thinks they are undescended.

If you have the birth record and the testes were found at that time, then you know there isn't a problem and can explain this to the parents. If not, then you have to find them yourself. Actually, this isn't too difficult with practice. Warm hands and a warm disposition help. I have prevented a number of children from having unnecessary operations in this way. A few years ago, a national study showed that about 70 per cent of operations to bring down an undescended testes were not necessary.

FRANCO

Franco was an eight-year-old boy whom I was asked to see because of suspected precocious puberty. His parents, Julietta and Guido Falcone, had noticed that he was developing early signs of puberty when he was seven years old.

Franco came to my clinic in a confident mood. He sat down, fixed me with a withering stare and said, 'Mum and Dad think I'm growing up too quickly.'

'And are you?' I asked him.

'I don't think so,' he said, firmly. 'I am about as big as my friends at school, though they think I'm a bit more muscly. Anyway, it's quite a good thing, 'cos I'm better at football than most of them.' This slight non sequitur put me in my place.

'Okay,' I said, 'Let me read this letter from your doctor.'

Franco settled down.

Guido and Julietta were Italian, having migrated from Italy ten years earlier, to work in a bistro owned by Julietta's uncle Marco. After five years, Marco had retired to Italy. He was unmarried and handed over the bistro to Julietta and Guido to run. By that time, they had three children, Franco, Carla, who was eleven and Margareta, seven. They lived in a large apartment that was over the bistro.

The GP said that Guido and Julietta had been concerned about Franco's development from quite an early age. Guido thought Franco was rather weedy and was keen to build him up through a good diet. Obviously, they were in a strong position to do so. They had taken him to the family doctor several times about this. As Franco became older, these anxieties seemed to lessen. When he was six, they had noticed that his penis was growing more than they had expected and took him to the practice again. Their GP had reassured them. However, over a period of a year or so, it had continued to grow until, recently, she had noticed the appearance of pubic hair. As there hadn't been any other signs of precocious puberty up until that point, such as an accelerated increase in his height, she hadn't been worried, but wanted another opinion.

The story was a little unusual, I thought.

I took a history, but, at this point, nothing turned up.

'Please may I examine you?'

'Okay.'

Franco was a well-developed boy for his age, but his growth was within the appropriate limits for that of his parents. However, his penis was significantly large for his age and he showed the development of a significant amount of pubic hair. Something was definitely amiss.

'I agree with you,' I said. 'His sexual development is a bit early. We need to investigate him to find out whether Franco has started to produce the hormones that trigger the onset of puberty early. I will arrange for the tests and we'll meet again to go through the results.'

Checking for the causes of precocious puberty involve several different tests and X-rays, so we arranged for some timed collections of urine at home, blood tests taken at suitable moments and X-rays of his bone maturity.

A few weeks later, they returned to my clinic.

'Well,' I said. 'Franco's results are a bit mixed. On the one hand, there are signs that he is developing a bit early, such as his bone maturity is a little advanced, though not a lot. But there doesn't seem to be any significant change in the levels of his pubertal hormones. On our stimulus tests, though, they do go up rather quickly.'

I decided, fortunately, to explore Franco's history a bit more.

'When Franco was quite young, you were both concerned that his physical development was inadequate, I'm told. Is that right?'

'Yes,' said Guido. 'We took him to Dr Blatch, but she said he was fine. So, we tried to build him up and, eventually, managed to help him.'

'This was with the excellent food in your bistro, I suppose.'

'To begin with, but that wasn't quite enough. Eventually, we started him on a tonic and that seemed to do the trick.'

'What tonic is that?'

'Pranzo!' Guido announced. I wasn't sure whether he'd sneezed, or that he thought I had.

'What's that?'

'It's an Italian tonic that my mother recommended,' said Julietta.

'Do you know what's in it?'

'Not really,' she admitted.

I thought this deserved further investigation. I arranged to meet them again in a week, by which time I planned to know all about Pranzo.

After searching carefully, I discovered that Pranzo, which means lunch in Italian, contained both cyproheptadine, an antihistamine that can cause adrenal suppression, and methandienone, which is a testosterone analogue than can cause virilisation. It was heavily marketed in Italy as an appetite stimulant. Here was the cause.

We met again.

'It turns out,' I began, cautiously, not wanted to cast a slur upon granny, 'that the medicines in Pranzo can cause the side effects that we have seen in the development of Franco's signs of puberty. That's good. If we just stop giving it to him, the changes present won't regress, but they won't progress until the right time.'

'It would be a good idea to let your mother know about this,' I said to Mrs Falcone, 'to protect her other grandchildren.'

'Oh yes,' she said.

All was well after that.

SANDRA

Sandra was a twelve-year-old who I was asked to see by one of my obstetric colleagues. She was pregnant, but was not forthcoming about how this pregnancy had occurred. The reason for the referral was that, when she had presented to my colleague six months through her pregnancy, a vaginal discharge had been noticed and swabbed. Culture of the swab revealed the presence of the gonococcus. She had begun treatment for this, but it was important to find out from whom Sandra had acquired her gonorrhoea.

I sat down with Sandra and her mother, Rheanna in the obstetric clinic in mid-October.

'Hello,' I began. 'How are you?'

'I'm all right,' said Sandra. 'Just a bit fed up by all the questioning.'

'I have been told that your baby is fine.'

'Yes, it's all going well, apparently,' said Rheanna. 'School have set her work to do at home and a friend collects it every day on her way. She brings back the next lot on her way home.' She seemed surprisingly unworried by her daughter's condition.

This was long before the Internet age and online school as we now know it.

'It must be a bit boring, doing it all your own and not seeing your friends.'

'Yes, but I'm going back in a week.'

'Good. Did you have a good holiday this summer?'

'Yes, we went to Southend for a week,' said Sandra. 'It was nice, but not as good as our Easter one.'

'Tell me about that.'

'I visited my cousins in Chicago. I had a lovely time.'

'On your own?'

'Yes,' said Rheanna. 'We couldn't all afford to go, so Sandra went with her older sister Susan. She's twenty.'

'What did you do when you were there?' I asked, trying to look as though this was an innocent question.

'Oh, we went out a lot.'

'Sightseeing?'

'A bit, but mostly in the evening, 'cos I have been before. We went to clubs and things.'

'Aren't you a bit young?'

'I was with Susan and she and her cousins managed to get me in with them. No one really checks much.'

'Meet anyone interesting?'

'Oh yes, lots of people.'

'Anyone special?'

'Only Tyrone, but he doesn't really count. He's a second cousin and lives next door in Chicago.'

'How old is he?'

'Ten, I think.'

'What did you do with Tyrone?'

'Oh, we got really close. He's really nice and has lots of girlfriends.'

I was getting an uncomfortable feeling about this. I turned to Rheanna.

'Have you any idea how Sandra got in the family way?'

'No, she won't tell me. Having babies early is common in our family.'

Really, I thought, twelve is a bit too early. But I didn't like to say so, given Rheanna's nonchalance.

'Aren't you worried about Sandra's gonorrhoea?' I asked.

'Yes, I was,' said Rheanna, 'but she's on treatment now.' That seemed to be okay, as far as she was concerned.

I tried to get a name from Sandra, without success.

'Well,' I said to Rheanna. 'I think the best we can do is to follow this up with your brother and his wife in Chicago. Can you do that? It's not very likely, but ask them to check out Tyrone as well, though he's a bit young.'

'All right,' she replied.

'Give me a ring if you get anything useful from them.' I gave her my number.

The next afternoon she phoned me in a great state.

'Oh dear,' she said. 'Apparently Tyrone hasn't been well. They discovered that he had a discharge, took him to the doctor last week and he's got gonorrhoea too! He's on treatment now.'

'Have you asked Sandra whether she had sex with him?'

'First thing I did. She admitted that she had, but swore that no one else was involved. I believe her.'

It eventually turned out that an aunt had introduced Tyrone

to sex, which was where he'd picked up gonorrhoea.

Although twelve is young for a girl to have a baby, Tyrone remains the youngest boy I have ever come across to have had sexual intercourse and produced a baby as a result. Little Vincent was born healthy and remains well, so far as I know.

5.

Bones and Joints

GENEVIEVE

When a young person develops arthritis that needs serious treatment, it is critically important to manage them especially carefully. Damage to a joint at a young age can cause deformities that disable them through life. We owe an enormous debt to the late Dr Barbara Ansell, who laid the foundations of optimal care for these children.

Genevieve Bingham came to my clinic complaining of joint pains. The letter from her GP described how, from being a twelve-year-old keen on sport, as well as academically bright, she had been compelled to give up many activities, because of pain. She was accompanied by her mother, Sylvia. Sylvia and her husband Bob ran a bookshop. She had a librarian's serious demeanour and wore her hair in a tight bun.

'When did you first start getting painful joints?' I asked.

'It must have been nearly a year ago, but I didn't pay too much attention at the time. I just thought I'd overdone things and injured myself at hockey.'

'Which were the painful ones?'

'It started in my knees, then, gradually, it's involved my hips, my hands and sometimes my feet.'

'Have you noticed anything else?'

'I've had some joint swelling and they have been warm to the touch. I've had a slight pinkish rash on my shins and forearms.'

This sounded very much like the onset of juvenile idiopathic arthritis (JIA). This is a condition that we needed to control quickly, in order to minimise the risk of joint damage. I took a full history. There was an aunt in Ireland who suffered from rheumatoid arthritis and possibly another relation with it in the Midlands, but they weren't sure about that. There was nothing else of significance.

'May I have a look at you?'

'Of course.'

I examined Genevieve. She was, in general, a healthy girl. She was a faint rash of tiny pinkish dots on her forearms and her shins. Her hip joint had a range of movement limited by pain, especially on the right. There was thickening of the synovia (the linings of her joints) of her fingers and her knees. Her grip was limited by pain when she squeezed my fingers.

'Well, as you thought, you have arthritis. We'll need to do some tests, to see which kind of arthritis you have and how active it is. I think we should start you on some treatment in the meantime, just a non-steroidal anti-inflammatory medicine until we get your results. After that, we will probably need to give you something to try to make it go away.'

I wasn't very hopeful, as this looked like the sort of arthritis that would go on for a long time.

Her results came back. She was 'sero-positive'; in other words, she had a juvenile form of rheumatoid arthritis. Her inflammatory markers showed that her disease was quite active.

She returned to the clinic early; she was in a lot of pain.

One characteristic of JIA is that the disease can flare up from time to time. This was one such flare. In particular, the pain in her right hip was a lot worse. She was limping.

'We need to start you on some steroids, to bring this flare under control. As you know, steroids are quite powerful and have a lot of side effects. I'll start you on a fairly high dose, but, as soon as you're better, we'll taper it off and, if necessary, put you on a dose every other day. This minimises the side effects while controlling your arthritis.'

'What if the steroids don't agree with me?'

'We'll cross that bridge when we come to it, but there are other treatments we can introduce, if we need to.'

We set off on a period of therapeutic trial. The prednisolone, her steroid, worked well, but, over a period of months, she couldn't reduce her alternate day steroid treatment without her joint flaring up again. We had another discussion.

'I think we ought to start you on methotrexate,' I said. 'This is an anti-cancer drug, but it can be very good at controlling arthritis. I think it would give you a good chance of coming off steroids and being pain free.'

'All right, let's try it,' said Genevieve.

Methotrexate was a great success. Not only did Genevieve have no flare-ups, but also she was able to enjoy her sports again.

After two years, her arthritis was controlled by a fairly low dose of methotrexate and she was now sixteen years old. It was time to transfer her care to the adult rheumatologists. We had a joint handover clinic with them. We said our goodbyes.

A year later, I had a phone call from her.

'What's the problem?' I asked.

'I'm walking like a duck!' she exclaimed. 'May I come and see you?'

'Of course.'

When she turned up, she was limping badly.

'What treatment are you on?' I asked.

'Just anti-inflammatory drugs,' she said, surprisingly. I had stressed the importance of maintaining her treatment to the rheumatology team. What had changed?

I examined Genevieve's joints. To my horror, her right leg was now 2 cm shorter than her left leg. No wonder she was limping.

It turned out that her care had been delegated to a relatively inexperienced registrar. He had decided that, as her joints were in such good shape, she didn't need to be on methotrexate, so had stopped it. Soon afterwards, Genevieve had a major flare-up, but still he gave neither steroids nor methotrexate.

I admit I was furious. Her tests showed lots of inflammatory changes. I gave her a short course of prednisolone, to bring her arthritis under control, and restarted her methotrexate.

It was too late, of course. The 2-cm loss in her right leg was permanent. Genevieve had to have a lift in her shoes to compensate.

The rheumatologist was apologetic and took over her care himself. It didn't help; the damage had been done.

PAMELA

Pamela Urquhart was thirteen. She had been limping on and off for about six weeks. Her family doctor though that her right hip was painful, but he couldn't find anything else wrong with her. He wondered whether this was the result of a hockey injury, as she was a keen sportswoman. He had given her an anti-inflammatory drug, ibuprofen, which had helped a bit, but it wasn't getting any better.

Pamela limped into my clinic with her mother, Patience. She sat down with a sigh. She was dressed in her school uniform, which consisted of a rather ugly yellow tartan pleated skirt and a white blouse with a black blazer. She shifted uncomfortably.

'I can see your hip's painful,' I said.

'Yes,' she said, 'and my uniform is ghastly too. This skirt is very itchy!'

'She's always complaining about it,' said Mrs Patience Urquhart. She was a stocky lady in a blouse and a pleated skirt.

'Apart from your hip,' I asked Pamela, 'is anything else painful?'

'Not really,' she said. 'My fingers hurt sometimes, but I think that's when I have a lot of writing to do. And I'm a bit stiff when I get up in the morning.'

'Oh dear,' I said. 'Does the stiffness last all day?'

'No,' said Pamela. 'It wears off after a while. Then it starts hurting again later.'

'Is that a different sort of pain?'

'Yes.'

I took a careful history. All was normal. Then I asked,

'Anyone in the family have skin problems?'

'No,' said Pamela.

'We've a Scottish aunt whose supposed to suffer with her skin, but I don't know what it is. She has another relative with the same problem. I can find out,' said Patience.

'All right. But let's see what's wrong here first. May I examine you, Pamela?'

'All right.' She got onto the examination couch with some difficulty.

I looked at her hands, often a good start. Then I looked more closely.

'Have you noticed these?' I said, pointing at her fingernails.

'No, what?' said Pamela.

'Can you see these tiny holes in your nails, like little pinpricks?'

'Oh yes,' she said. 'Look at these, Mum. What are they?'

'I'll tell you in a minute.'

I looked at her fingers. Some of the joints were a bit swollen and Pamela winced a little when I flexed and extended those fingers. I examined her other joints. Her right hip movement was restricted by pain, but her other large joints were normal. I looked in her hair. There was a small red flaky patch near the nape of her neck.

'What's this?' I asked.

'It's just a rash I've got. Mum has been putting E45 on it.'

The rest of her examination was normal.

'I think your problem is something called psoriasis.'

'But I thought that gave you lots of scaly skin. I didn't think children got it. I have a friend who has it,' said Mrs Urquhart.

'Yes, that's true,' I replied. 'But it can occur in children. The clues are the little pits in your fingernails. They are typical of psoriasis. And psoriasis can cause arthritis, particularly affecting the sort of joints that are bothering you. I think your finger problems are due to it and the patch of scaly skin on your neck is a little psoriatic one.'

'Can you make me better?' Pamela asked.

'Oh yes,' I said confidently. 'We need to carry out some tests to see what sort of condition you're in and whether there are any confirmatory results. In the meantime, I will increase your dose of ibuprofen, which is nowhere near enough to help your arthritis. If that isn't effective, we can give you something that will work better. I'll ask one of our children's skin specialists to advise about your scaly patch too.'

I arranged for Pamela to have some blood tests and an X-ray of her hips. It was early in her arthritis, so the hips looked normal, fortunately. Her blood tests showed raised inflammatory markers and positive anti-nuclear antibody, sometimes seen in children with psoriatic arthritis.

Her arthritis proved quite difficult to control, which is not uncommon in this condition. In the end, we put her on methotrexate, like Genevieve. That helped a lot and she remained pain-free until we transferred her care to the adult rheumatologists.

BENJAMIN

Benjamin was an eighteen-month-old toddler who had stopped walking. His GP told me that not only was he refusing to walk now, having begun to do so about four or five months earlier, but he wasn't keen on sitting either. Mrs Muriel Keen, his mother, was propping him up for his meals, but he now preferred to lie down, in which position he seemed to be happier.

They arrived in the clinic, Ben was in a pushchair and was cheerful.

'When did this happen?' I inquired.

'One morning about three weeks ago,' said Muriel Keen. 'After breakfast I took him to play in the living room, but all he wanted to do was to sit on the floor and play with his toys. Up until then, he'd been toddling about collecting his toys and playing with them. For a week or two he went back to bottom-shuffling, but then he wouldn't do that either. For the last few days, he only sits reluctantly, so I have had him in an angled seat, which he seems to like.'

'Can he tell you what he feels is wrong?'

'Yes, he used to be quite chatty but less so now. When I ask him if he wants to walk, he just says, "No", but when I ask him why, he just says, "Don't want to". I asked him if it hurts and he says, "Don't know". Not very helpful, I know!'

'Do you think it's a muscle or a nerve problem? Can he move his arms and legs all right?'

'Yes, they seem normal. If I pick him up, he feels just the same. If he doesn't want to be picked up, he struggles in the way he always did. I don't think it's a movement problem.'

'Have you any idea what you think it might be?' This is a crucial question. As I've said earlier, mothers' observations are key to unravelling a mysterious problem, indeed any medical problem in children. They may not know what it is, but what they notice is very important.

'No, I haven't a clue. I almost feel he's just being difficult, but I know it can't be that, because he's been much too consistent. I'd expect his behaviour to change from day to day and it hasn't, it's just got worse. It must be something wrong with him, I'm sure.'

I thought this was an astute observation. Whatever it was, it was organic. My SHO recited his medical history, as he'd seen him first. I asked a few supplementary questions. Dr Phillips described his examination, it was normal.

I took a look at Ben. I examined him neurologically and looked at his joints. They were all normal.

'The first things to do are some basic investigations: blood count, inflammatory markers, MSU (mid-stream urine microscopy and culture) and so on. When I have the results, we'll see him again next week.'

'What do you think is wrong with him?' asked Mrs Keen.

'I confess I really don't know, but I am certain that you're right, Ben has something going on. We will sort it out and, as he's generally well otherwise, I think we can do this as an outpatient.'

'Thank you,' she said.

Two days later Ben's results arrived on my desk. His inflammatory markers were raised and he had a high left-shifted neutrophil count. This strongly suggested that he had an infection of some sort. But where? His urine culture and microscopy were normal and his upper respiratory system, including his ears, and his chest were clear. Dr Phillips and I had a conference.

'I'll phone Mrs Keen today and ask her to bring him back. I think, under the circumstances, we ought to admit him for a few days. We must find out where this infection is. I'll let you know when he's coming' I said.

Ben was admitted and I saw him again. There was still nothing to find clinically, though he did now have a low-grade fever, which he hadn't had in the clinic.

'As I said when we spoke on the phone, we need to find where this infection is. We'll do a blood culture and, I think, it would be worth doing a bone scan. Sometimes a bone infection can be quiet clinically. There's nothing to suggest meningitis, so we'll wait on doing a lumbar puncture, but keep it up our sleeve.'

The tests were arranged. Next morning, after the bone scan, the paediatric nuclear medicine consultant rang me.

'It's difficult to be sure because, in kids of this age there's so much growing going on at the bone ends, a lot shows up on the scan. But I think there's a hotter spot at T11 (the eleventh thoracic vertebra). I'll send you the films.'

I had a look, T11 did show up on the films more strongly than its neighbours. I had a chat with the paediatric orthopaedic team.

'Can you carry out a needle biopsy of this vertebra?' I showed them the pictures.

'We could, but it would be tricky.'

'Shall we wait for the blood culture? That might help us,' I suggested.

'All right. If that's positive, then we could postpone the biopsy.'

The microbiologist rang me next morning.

'We've got a Strep faecalis in Benjamin Keen's blood culture. Is that helpful?'

'Yes,' I said thankfully. We could be sure that Ben had vertebral osteomyelitis. This is an organism found in the gut and usually doesn't cause much in the way of disease. Its character explained why Ben wasn't as toxically ill as one might have expected. It explained why he didn't like walking or standing. It hurt!

We started Ben on a six-week course of antibiotics. This wasn't much fun for him as, in order to make sure it was effective, it had to be given intravenously. However, with the help of the excellent community paediatric nursing team and the presence of a series of intravenous cannulae left *in situ* for a few days each, he was able to be at home.

Two weeks after he started his treatment, Ben was walking again.

6.

Parents Can Be Different

PETER

Peter was a happy six-year-old who trotted obediently into my clinic with his mother and younger sister. They concentrated on the play area, where Susie, his sister, led them in a complicated game of families.

Peter's GP letter was clear. 'Peter is a contented little boy who has been making steady progress in his first year at school. He is very well behaved, but his teachers have found that he is little slower than the other children. His mother, Mrs Davis, says that, in retrospect, he was slower than his sister to learn to speak and to walk, but not dramatically. I can't see anything obviously wrong with him and I would be grateful for your opinion.'

While the two children played, Peter's mother and I chatted. Emily Davis was well dressed and dark haired. She worked as a dental hygienist. One dentist in the practice was her husband Dai. She wasn't unduly worried about Peter. Her pregnancy and Peter's birth had been uncomplicated and he had passed all the checks that were carried out on him. He didn't walk until he was eighteen months old and his first words were a little earlier. He hadn't had any significant illnesses, though Mrs Davis thought he became breathless more easily than his sister. He had made lots of friends at school and was popular.

Taken together, the story indicated a child who was mildly developmentally delayed. The question was why.

On looking at Peter while he played, there were obvious family resemblances. However, his face was a little flatter than one would have expected, his ears were a little small and, significantly, his palpebral fissures – in other words the spaces within which his eyes sat – showed a very slight upwards slant towards his ears.

I called him over and sat him on the couch. When I lifted him up, he was a little floppier than I would have expected, suggesting that his muscle tone was slightly low. He smiled at me. Most of the physical examination was normal. However, on listening to his chest, I could hear a soft heart murmur in the middle of systole, the period when the main chambers of the heart are contracting. I could also hear the sounds of the heart valves opening and closing and that the second heart sound had a fixed split. This sound is caused by the closure of two heart valves and the gap between the two noises normally varies as the child breathes in and out. In Peter's case the split between the two noises didn't vary. The murmur and the fixed split suggested that he had an atrial septal defect. On looking at his chest again, I noticed that, when he breathed in more deeply, there was 'intercostal recession': the spaces between his ribs was sucked in slightly. This observation fitted in nicely, as it implied that his lungs were a little stiffer than normal.

I looked at Peter's hands. Normally, there are two main skin creases across the palm. In his case, there was only one on each hand. The diagnosis was clear.

'Mrs Davis,' I began. 'I will need to carry out one or two tests, but I think the reasons for Peter's mild slowness are because he has an abnormality of his chromosomes. For several reasons, I think this abnormality is heterogeneous. Put another way, I don't think it affects all the cells in his body, although probably a majority of them. I think the affected cells have an extra copy of chromosome 21. This is the cause of Down Syndrome, but in Peter's case I suspect he has what we would call Mosaic Down Syndrome, because only some of his cells are affected.'

Mrs Davis became visibly upset, but did her best to hold things together so as not to upset her children.

I continued. 'Many children like Peter do as well as their peers at school, though it sounds as though he is a bit slower. However, I don't think this will be a big problem and with additional educational support he is likely to hold his own. He does need to have a few tests.'

'What sort of tests? Will he need any treatment? Will he have to go to a special school?'

Mrs Davis was going through an experience that most parents have when confronted by a stressful diagnosis. A plethora of questions come into their heads and they often ask them in no sort of logical order. It's best to wait until they pause for breath.

'First of all, we need to check his chromosomes. We need to

see that his thyroid hormone levels are normal, as some children with this condition can have low levels. The chromosomal problems also often lead to heart abnormalities. I think Peter has a small hole between the two smaller heart chambers, the atria. This is allowing rather more blood to flow through his lungs with each heartbeat. This makes his lungs a bit stiffer and is probably the reason he gets a bit more breathless than Susie when they run about. If I am right, it can probably be closed quite easily and without needing a major heart operation. Often, the heart specialists can pass a catheter through the hole and open a sort of double-sided umbrella that will close it off. Quite straightforward.'

Our discussion continued for a while and the children went on playing. Peter's investigations revealed that he did have a Mosaic Down Syndrome, some 60 per cent of his cells having Trisomy 21. He had an atrial septal defect, which was closed *via* a catheter. He did not have hypothyroidism.

He made steady progress at school, passing most of his exams. He decided to take up teaching and now works in a primary school. He has married and, together with his wife, they have decided upon artificial insemination by donor (AID).

JEAN

Fourteen-year-old Jean came to see me because her mother was concerned that she wasn't yet showing any sign of entering puberty. The letter from Dr Moss, her GP, said that Jean was a shy young lady who was quite healthy, but, as he put rather quaintly, who was not yet developing any signs of womanhood.

'It's about time,' said Maureen MacMillan, her mother. 'I have two older girls and they all went through puberty between about eleven and thirteen, so we're not slow in our family.'

Jean looked rather embarrassed by all this. She was slim and of slightly less than average height for her age.

'Have you had any problems or illnesses in the past?' I asked Jean, trying to centre the discussion around her.

'No, she's always been a healthy young lady. Just coughs and colds, you know. No visits to hospital and none to our doctor, apart from the routine ones.' Mrs MacMillan was a formidable woman.

Further discussion failed to reveal anything of interest.

I carried out a complete physical examination. There was absolutely nothing to give me a hint that anything was wrong. Apart from one thing. While I was checking that there really were no signs of puberty – there weren't – I noticed two small lumps in her groins, one on either side. They were a little too low down to be lymph nodes, just in the upper level of the labia majora. I wondered.

'Jean, so far as I can tell, you are entirely a healthy young lady. Certainly, you aren't entering puberty. Tell, me, those two small lumps we found, had you noticed them before.'

'Yes,' she said.

'When was that?' I asked.

'Oh, a long time ago.'

'More than a year?'

'Yes, much more.'

Interesting, I thought.

'Jean, I think we should do one or two tests, just to see that everything is as it should be. Is that all right with you?'

'I suppose so.' Mrs MacMillan was, fortunately, silent.

'It'll mean a blood test and a ultrasound test, to see whether we can identify what your two little lumps are.'

'When will that be?' asked Mrs McMillan.

'We can do the blood test today and the ultrasound in a week or so. Shall we meet after that?'

'All right.'

I waited for the results of Jean's investigations, in some trepidation. Unfortunately, my guess seemed to be correct. We met in the clinic again.

'Hello, are you still well?' I asked Jean, nervously.

'What did my tests show?' she asked, quickly.

'Well, most of them are quite normal, apart from the chromosomal test we did and the ultrasound.'

'What did they show?'

'The chromosome test showed that you have twenty-two paired chromosomes, plus an X and a Y chromosome. The ultrasound test showed that your two little lumps are two small testes.'

'Do you mean that Jean's a boy?' demanded Mrs MacMillan, angrily.

'Not exactly. I think Jean has a condition called complete testicular feminisation syndrome. It means that, although she has the chromosomes of a boy, the cells in her body don't have a working version of a receptor for testosterone, the main male hormone. Because of this, when she was developing as a fetus, her body couldn't undergo the changes that would turn her into a boy. When that happens, the children that are born like this all look like girls. We would say that they have a male genotype, but a female phenotype.'

'What can we do now?'

'That will need a lot of discussion. Effectively, there is no reason why Jean shouldn't continue to identify as a girl. If so, I would recommend that the two small testes should be removed, as they carry a small risk of developing into a cancer if we leave them there. If you'd rather be a boy, Jean, that would be a more complicated process and would mean a bit more surgery.'

'I'm sure she should stay as a girl, so can she have babies?'

'Unfortunately not, but that's one of the things we need to discuss with her.'

This was going to be tricky, as Mrs MacMillan's wishes must be subordinate to Jean's.

'We have some special counsellors who are trained to help with this sort of situation. I would recommend that Jean meet one of them. After that, she can decide what else to do.'

I set up the meeting with one of these counsellors, who I knew would ensure that Jean's views would be heard and adhered to. As it happened, Jean couldn't think of being anything but a girl, so her redundant testes were removed.

I never saw her again, but I heard, some fifteen years later, that she had trained as a nurse, got married and had adopted two children.

ELLIOTT

Advances in the screening of the fetus for abnormality has brought with it a host of problems in supporting parents when abnormality is discovered.

David and Sally Briggs were a British couple who had trained and practiced as physiotherapists in London. After a time, they emigrated to America and built up a successful business there, treating a variety of physical problems.

Eventually, they decided it was time to start a family and, soon afterwards, Sally became pregnant. Being aware of the problems that might lie ahead, Sally invested in high quality antenatal care. At her first ten-week scan, she was alerted to the probability that her baby had an abnormality of the spine. A repeat scan, soon afterwards, confirmed that her baby, a boy, had a form of spinal abnormality know as spinal rachischisis. This is a more severe form of spina bifida, in which the spinal cord remains opened out flat over the unfused vertebrae of the lower back.

The Briggs were devastated. They were aware of the US legislation on these matters, framed in California by the 'Baby Doe' case. They were strongly in favour of aborting their child, but this meant that they would be unable to do so in America. Furthermore, even if they returned to the UK, it would be too late to obtain one, as Sally's pregnancy was, by now, too far advanced.

They decided to return anyway, because they believed that it would be easier in the UK to ensure that a severely damaged newborn baby could be allowed to pass away without the application of resuscitation, should he fail to breathe normally after birth.

When they returned, they arranged to see an obstetrician colleague of mine. He asked that I join him for the initial consultation, having been made aware of the situation.

The four of us had a long discussion. Sally agreed that her pregnancy, which was progressing normally, should go to term. However, she asked me to promise that, under no circumstances would I resuscitate her baby, but allow him to die. This was something I could not promise to do, but I managed to satisfy her by saying, somewhat mendaciously, that I wouldn't interfere with her son's immediate postnatal progress. However, I insisted that, if he was distressed, I would need to act to relieve him. Of course, this might well mean supporting his breathing, but I managed to avoid pointing this out. Mrs Briggs agreed, because she didn't want him to suffer in any way.

Labour duly arrived and their son, Elliott, was born. I made sure that I was present at his delivery, rather than a member of our on-call paediatric team. He was an active baby boy, who needed no intervention from me and began to breathe, and to yell, swiftly. Apart from the paralysis of his lower limbs as a consequence of his spinal abnormality, he was entirely healthy.

There followed a four-day period of uncertainty. The correct procedure would have been to take Elliott to surgery as soon as possible and to close the open spinal cord on his back. However, his parents did not want this done, initially, probably because they were finding it hard to decide what best to do. Outside, my paediatric surgical colleague was champing at the bit. Not the most patient of men, though a brilliant surgeon, he harangued me regularly, wanting to get his hands on Elliott. I had my work cut out keeping him away from the Briggs, because I knew that his aggressive approach might drive them over the edge and Elliott might not get his operation.

After four days of gentle listening and persuasion, Sally Briggs agreed that Elliott should have surgery. He was doing very well by then. Everything went smoothly and soon they were able to fly back to America, apprehensive about what lay ahead.

I received regular reports from the Briggs about Elliott. Gradually they came, first, to accept his disability and, as time passed, to become the proud parents of a boy who grew into a remarkable wheelchair-bound young man. Although he developed the complications we had anticipated, needing a Spitz-Holter valve to relieve his developing hydrocephalus and having recurrent urinary tract infections, he did well academically, graduating from university and is now practising as a family lawyer.

PAUL

Occasionally I would ask students in my clinic what they noticed about my consultations. Sometimes, one might say 'I thought you were a bit waffly at the beginning.'

'Yes,' I would reply. 'Can you think why that might be?' Various reasons would be offered, usually wrong!

'I do it deliberately,' I would say. 'I have never met this family before and I need to know what they are like and what their beliefs and, indeed, their prejudices are. It's very important to do this, so as to structure the consultation and my responses to them to ensure that a strong relationship is formed and they feel able to trust me. If I say the wrong thing, I could lose their support for ever.'

Sometimes, however hard you try, your relationship with the parents is doomed before it has even begun.

Paul was a newborn baby who had obvious congenital abnormalities. He was of low birthweight, had a small head, abnormalities of his hands and feet, small malformed ears and was extremely difficult to feed. Neither we, not our clinical genetic colleagues, could fit him into a known congenital syndrome, though we sent off his chromosomes for investigations.

He was transferred into my care for further investigations and treatment. His main problem was his feeding. He would start to feed, then stop and scream in such a way as to suggest he was in pain. We were having to feed him slowly by nasogastric tube.

After further examination and thought, my opinion was that he had a serious cardiac abnormality. I sent him to my paediatric cardiology colleagues for various investigations. They sent him back saying his heart was normal.

I didn't believe them, so I sent him to another paediatric cardiac team at a different hospital. They sent him back with the same answer. I still didn't believe them.

Fortunately, I had some helpful colleagues. I set up our own investigations. It emerged that Paul had complex congenital heart disease. He had two problems which, putting things simply, meant that, when Paul fed, his swallowing ability was restricted and, in addition, he was developing heart muscle pain – angina, in other words.

A relatively simple operation would abolish his pain and Paul would have been able to feed more comfortably. To arrange this, I needed his parents' consent.

After my initial examination, my first action had been to sit down and discuss him with his parents. I described his multiple abnormalities to them and said that we would do our best to find out what was wrong with his feeding, so that he could thrive better. However, I added the caveat that his underlying genetic condition was most probably untreatable. At this point, his parents seemed to accept the plan.

I met them again, in order to explain the situation. His parents, George and Clarissa Stevens, were the blonde, blue-eyed paragons of a wealthy family. George worked in a bank, Clarissa did lots of 'good works'. They had a lovely blonde, blue-eyed daughter of four called Amanda. Paul was meant to be the blonde, blue-eyed boy to complete their perfect family. They were living presently in Dubai, but had returned for Paul's birth in our private wing.

I told them that Paul needed a small operation, to improve his quality of life and I asked them whether they had any questions about this.

'How long do you think he will live?' asked George, rather abruptly.

'That's difficult to say,' I replied. 'Our first job is to give him the best quality of life we can, so that he is as contented as we can make him. After that we will see, though my guess, at this point, is that he isn't likely to survive a long time.'

'Isn't there something you can do to make sure that he doesn't suffer for too long?' asked Clarissa.

'Well, that's what I am working on,' I replied.

I was now becoming rather worried. I wasn't sure what Paul's parents were thinking about and I needed their help and support.

'Are you willing to give your permission for Paul to have this operation?' I asked.

'Can you give us some time to think about it?' George replied.

'Of course,' I said, 'But I would like an answer by tomorrow, if possible.' They agreed.

They left and I went back to the ward. The nursing staff were desperate for Paul to have his surgery, because they could feel the pain he was in. They were disappointed by the delay.

They next day I received a note from the Stevens, in which they said that they wouldn't give permission for Paul to have surgery.

I went to see Paul. Both his grandmothers were at his cot. They asked me what was happening. I explained the situation.

'Oh, they are impossible!' declared George's mother. 'I'm not surprised they refused consent. They have been saying the most upsetting things to us about Paul.'

'Yes,' said Clarissa's mum. 'We have been appalled by their seeming heartlessness. We have, obviously, discussed it amongst the family. Everyone else wants Paul to have this operation, but his parents aren't convinced it's the best thing.'

'I would be very grateful if you can do your best to persuade them,' I said. They said they would.

Our entire team, especially the nurses caring for him, was distressed. My only option was to make Paul a Ward of Court and take it out of his parents' hands. After some discussion with my colleagues and the team, we decided, against our better judgement, to give Paul's parent a chance to change their minds. I spoke with them and was blunt.

'Paul needs this operation, not to save his life, but to make his life tolerable. I am going on a week's annual leave. If you still refuse to give permission for surgery, we will undertake proceedings to make Paul a Ward of Court.'

The Stevens were angry about this, but other than removing him from my care, there was little they could do. Clearly, they couldn't take him home and, if they tried, they would have to sign a form saying they were removing him against medical advice. Should then he pass away in a day or so, they would be in a very weak position.

I went on leave, asking my colleagues not to allow him to be discharged.

I returned a week later. Paul had gone. A colleague of mine *had* allowed his transfer to another, private hospital and Paul died on his first day there. I was very upset, but there was nothing more I could do.

Some three months later I went abroad on sabbatical for a year. While I was there, I received a letter from one of my colleagues. Apparently, George Stevens had been threatening to write an official letter of complaint about the way I had managed Paul's case. He asked me what I thought they should do about it.

I replied 'Do nothing. I think Mr and Mrs Stevens feel guilty about what happened to Paul and this is a way of passing off some of their guilt to me. They won't follow it up.'

We never heard from them again.

7.

Nappy and Other Rashes

Nappy rashes are the cause of lots of maternal anxiety. Sometimes the parents think it's some sort of allergy, or possibly they've been told it's 'baby eczema'. Mostly it's nothing like that.

Apart from rarities, there are, in my opinion, only three common kinds of nappy rash in babies. One is caused by ammonia released from urine, a second type by thrush, caused by the presence of a fungus called Candida albicans, and the third, which is a combination of the two.

They are easy to treat, too. If it's just ammoniacal dermatitis, all you have to do is sprinkle a few drops of vinegar onto the disposable nappy before you put it on the baby. That neutralises the ammonia and the rash disappears, often overnight. That caused by thrush should be treated by an ointment called Nystaform HC, a combination of the anti-fungal agent with 1 per cent hydrocortisone. If both types occur, you use both treatments.

Provided you've made the correct diagnoses, I found these to cure the problem in short order.

Infantile eczema is sometimes accompanied by a nappy rash, but that's easy to recognise, as there will be a rash or rashes elsewhere.

GAIL

Gail was a four-month-old girl who was admitted with a sudden episode of rash and breathlessness. This had happened after her first feed with artificial milk and Charlotte Spencer, her mother, had brought her straight to our Children's A&E. They had treated her for anaphylaxis and admitted her for observation.

'I can't understand it,' said Charlotte, who was a lawyer. 'She's never had any milk before, so why should she have an immediate reaction?'

'What was the milk you gave her?' I asked.

'SMA,' she said. 'I have been breastfeeding her exclusively until now, but was about to start giving her some more solid food – a rusk with some milk, as the baby clinic suggested. I thought of using breast milk, but this seemed easier.'

'She's never had anything else by mouth?'

'No.'

'Do you have a family history of allergy?'

'Well, yes, I do. When I was small, Mother said I was allergic to cow's milk, but I grew out of it by the time I was less than five. I only remember having cow's milk, myself.'

'Do you have milk nowadays?'

'Yes, on cereal, in tea and coffee and sometimes in other ways. It doesn't affect me'

'No other allergies?'

'I get mild hay fever in the Spring, but otherwise no.'

It was fairly obvious that Charlotte was atopic, in other words an allergic type.

Gail was, by now, quite fine.

'We need to find out what Gail reacted to and why, so we can make sure she's safe. We can take some blood tests now and she can go home. I'd like some from you too, please, for the purposes of comparison. I'll see you both in my clinic with the results in about two weeks. In the meantime, keep her on breast milk only.'

Something many don't seem to realise it that one can have potential allergy in one's circulation, but not necessarily show any symptoms. There weren't absolutely reliable ways to find this out on a blood test, but it was worth a try.

We met again two weeks later.

'I think we know what happened,' I said. 'Your blood contains immunoglobulin E that reacts with casein, the cow's milk protein. Gail acquired an allergy to cow's milk from you, probably during pregnancy, or possibly from your breast milk, as breast milk is stuffed full with cells from the immune system. Because you were able to drink milk without symptoms, in spite of that, Gail's immune system picked up the allergy and, when she drank a little cow's milk, reacted acutely to it.'

'What do we do?'

'It's not complicated. Keep Gail off cow's milk for the moment and stay off it yourself until you stop breastfeeding. There is a good chance that her allergy will eventually go away. Our dietician will advise you on safe milks that you can give her for the moment. I'll arrange for her to be followed up in our children's allergy clinic and they will check her allergic status from time to time. They'll let you know if and when it's safe to try cow's milk again.'

'My husband and I are planning to have another child. What can I do to make sure this can't happen again?'

'Simple,' I said. 'Stay off cow's milk as soon as you start to plan to have a child. If you stay off it during pregnancy and breastfeeding, the baby shouldn't have any problems. Make sure you introduce cow's milk after about eighteen months of age, or so.'

The paediatric allergy consultant told me later, that Gail was free of cow's milk allergy by the time she was about four years old.

SHONA

Shona was twelve when we first met. Her family doctor asked me to see her because she had developed lumps on her legs which were red, raised, about 2–4 cm across and sore. Initially, he thought they might be chilblains, but more appeared and, later, some developed on her arms and her face.

By the time she came to see me in the clinic, some of those on her legs had begun to break down and ulcerate. The district nurse had been dressing them, but one or two had become infected.

Shona was, as you might imagine, distressed by this and had been off school. There was nothing in her history to suggest a cause for the condition. She didn't have a fever, but complained that the lesions were sore. I looked to see whether I could find any evidence of involvement of other organs than her skin, but without success.

Dr Findlater thought it was an allergic reaction of some sort, but I wasn't convinced. It was certainly inflammatory, but we needed better evidence.

'Would you mind if Shona came into the ward for a couple of days? We need to see whether we can find out what this is and I can get a skin specialist to see her. Would you be happy with that, Shona?'

Shona and her mother, Sylvia Fraser, agreed.

When Shona came into the ward, we arranged some specific tests, looking for some less common conditions, such as systemic lupus erythematosus (SLE) polyarteritis nodosa (PAN), sarcoidosis and alpha-1 antitrypsin disease, amongst a number. The tests were all negative.

We were fortunate in that the main skin specialist hospital in Britain was on site and they had several consultants expert in children's skin diseases. Dr Jamieson came to see her.

'Interesting,' he said, enigmatically. 'I'm not sure what this is. Best thing would be to biopsy one of the lesions.'

'I agree,' I concurred. 'Closest thing seems to be Weber-Christian Disease (WCD), but it's vanishingly rare in children.'

'Yes,' he agreed. 'Hopefully, we get a clue from the histology.'

Dr Jamieson arranged for the skin biopsy, something dermatologists do a lot. The results came back.

'Interesting,' he reiterated. 'The biopsy shows inflammation, without any vasculitis, in the fatty layer of the skin. Looks very like WCD. However, Shona doesn't have involvement of any other system, which is odd.'

'Could it be a reflection of her being so young?' I asked.

'Possibly. Why don't we treat her for it and see what happens.'

We started her on some steroid therapy, standard for WCD. Her lesions started to regress, but rather slowly. Dr Jamieson and I met again.

'Could we try Cyclosporine A?' I asked.

'Worth a go,' he agreed.

We started it and, in a month, her lesions healed up.

'I still think it was a bizarre form of allergy,' said a colleague, gloomily. 'It'll come back when you stop her treatment.

'Maybe,' I said. 'I've no idea. We'll just have to see.'

Over the next five years, Shona's skin lumps, now defined as recurrent panniculitis, came and went. Every time, a combination of prednisolone (the steroid) and Cyclosporine A got rid of it for a few weeks or months, then it came back. However, the intervals got longer and, but the time she was eighteen, they stopped. Phew!

We tried all sorts of tests to see whether she was allergic to anything. She was, to a few things, but nothing that tied into her condition. It remained a mystery.

DERRICK

Sometimes, just the fear of allergy can lead to a problem. Derrick came to me when he was just over fifteen months old. His mother, Yvette Woollard, was worried that he wasn't walking yet. He was a fat, healthy baby who should have been toddling, but seemed to be happy just sitting.

'I am really worried,' said Yvette Woollard. 'He's a happy

baby, but he doesn't want to stand. I try, but he just sits down again.'

I started to take a history. He'd been born at our hospital and the pregnancy and delivery were normal.

'Did you breastfeed him?' I inquired.

'Oh yes, I still am. We have a strong family history of allergy, so I'm trying to keep him off cow's milk for the moment.'

'Does he eat what the rest of the family have?'

'Mostly, though, if he does, I mush it up. I give him his own diet, so as to avoid anything that he might become allergic to.'

'That could be a lot of things,' I said, sympathetically. 'So many things can induce an allergic response.'

'Oh, I know!' she exclaimed. 'I work in a library, so I have access to a lot of useful books on the subject. It helps me to work out what is safe for him.'

I began to tease out exactly what Derrick was having in his diet. It was very limited!

I started to examine him. I stood him up, supporting him. There was marked curvature of his legs at the knees. I felt them. Palpable swelling of his metaphyses – the ends of the long bones – was present. I completed his examination. Oh dear, I had to break the news.

'I think that Derrick's diet has been a bit too limited. He's developed rickets.'

Mrs Woollard was visibly upset.

'There's no need to worry, it's fairly easy to put right and he'll be running about very soon.'

We got together with the dieticians and, together with added oral vitamin D, worked out a diet that was acceptable to Mrs Woollard, but had the right nutrients. Derrick made a swift recovery.

Sometimes, 'A little learning is a dangerous thing'!

8.

Being Fat Isn't Always a
Lifestyle Choice

CHRISTIAN

Christian Liebermann was a boy of twelve whose care I sort
of inherited from a colleague on a different campus. He had
been seen in the clinic for several years on account of his being
overweight. My colleague had a special interest in endocrine
disorders, but had concluded that Christian's problem was
a combination of both an unsuitable diet and idleness. He
had implemented a programme of dietary supervision and
encouraged Christian to take up interest in some active sports.

Christian wasn't a sporty sort of boy. He saw himself as more
of a nerd, spending much of his time playing computer games.
He was a happy lad, who obviously thought this was a fuss
about nothing. He was clearly well above the weight for his age
and height. My colleague's interventions didn't seem to have
achieved much, I thought.

Although there was no referral letter, he had a fat file of
notes, which I went through diligently. There were very little
in the way of investigations, although one result caught my

eye, but meticulous records of his growth and lots of comments from the dieticians. They found it hard to understand why Christian's weight wasn't coming within the normal range.

Mrs Liebermann was of average weight and height. 'Dad's a big chap,' she said, helpfully.

'What does he eat most days?' I asked.

'He's very good,' Ethel Liebermann said. 'He sticks to what Angela says he should have.' Angela was his dietician. 'He has the odd treat, but nothing out of the ordinary and Angela says she can't understand how he keeps his weight up.'

'How is he coping at school?'

'He does all right. He is usually somewhere in the middle of the class. When we go to a parents' evening, they say he could work a bit harder, that he's a bit lazy, lots of boys can be that way. We can't really complain and he likes it at his school.'

This sounded very normal.

'May I have a look at you?' I asked Christian. He shrugged and climbed awkwardly onto the couch. I began to check him over.

Apart from his being a large boy, everything was normal. Then I checked his tendon reflexes. I got the impression that they were a little sluggish and took a fraction of a second longer to relax than I would have expected. However, I was a bit cautious, as the one investigation I had noted may have made me expect this to be the case.

'I have been looking at his old notes,' I began. 'There is one test he had a year or two ago that seemed to me not to be quite as I would have expected.'

'What was that?' asked Ethel.

'It's a hormone called TSH, or thyroid stimulating hormone. The level in Christian's blood is rather higher than normal, though not very much so.'

'What could that mean?'

'It's possible that Christian's thyroid gland isn't making enough of the active hormone it should. What we need to do next it to check it again and, this time, measure the levels of the various thyroid hormone in Christian's blood.'

'Oh no!' protested Christian. I could understand his reluctance to have more blood tests: he had large arms, so finding a vein would be more difficult than usual.

'What would be the effect of putting this right, if the test's still abnormal?' asked Ethel.

'In the first place, it might be the reason why Christian has trouble controlling his weight. Also, it may be that his performance, both at school academically and with respect to sports, could benefit. Let's see.'

Christian went off for his blood tests. A week or two later he returned to the clinic with the results.

'Well, your TSH is still elevated,' I reported. 'They show too that the levels of active thyroid hormones in your blood are lower than they should be, ideally.'

We had checked to see whether he was making an abnormal sort of thyroid hormone, which is seen in some metabolic thyroid disorders with a genetic basis, and whether he was making antibodies to his thyroid hormones. Neither seemed to be the case.

'Can you help him?' asked Ethel.

'I think we can. We'll start him on a small dose of thyroid hormone by mouth and build it up slowly, checking his TSH level until it falls into the normal range. That will let us know when we are giving him enough.'

Christian came to the clinic at regular intervals. Over a period of about three months, we managed to get his thyroid hormone and TSH levels into the normal range on a fairly low dose of thyroxine. We waited to see what would happen.

Christian lost weight, but slowly. After a year or so, he settled at a more acceptable weight, still above the average of his height, but in line with his father's build. Angela was happier.

His school performance improved dramatically. Christian was now in the top two or three in his class and really enjoying school. He had begun to like some sports, developing an interest in rugby, where he developed into a formidable prop forward.

There is controversy as to whether such borderline cases of hypothyroidism should be given treatment. Obviously, my colleague who had looked after Christian's care initially thought not. Sometimes, though, the proof of the pudding is in the eating!

ARCHIBALD AND BRIAN

Childhood obesity is one of the health obsessions of the age. In nearly every case, it is a product of inappropriate diet and insufficient physical activity. Once one has obtained a proper history, finding a solution is usually quite simple, but implementing it is another matter.

Archie and Brian were two unrelated children that I was asked to see on separate occasions. Their histories were remarkably similar, though Archie was five and Brian six. Interestingly, they were suffering from different conditions that happened to have almost identical effects upon them.

Archie was born in Croydon of healthy parents of a normal size. He had two older siblings, a brother two years older and a sister four years older. They were also healthy. His parents, Sylvia and George Thomas, realised that Archie was a bit different early on. He was always hungry and he put on weight at an alarming rate. They struggled to control his food intake and sought the help of their local paediatric and dietary services when he was in his second year.

A series of dietary modifications were tried and failed to help him. The paediatric team carried out a panoply of investigations, looking for hormonal and biochemical abnormalities and checking his genetic background. Everything was normal. They continued to monitor his growth, which continued relentlessly upwards.

I met his paediatrician at a regional meeting and heard about him.

'Would you like to see him?' she asked.

'If you would really like me to,' I said, reluctantly, not seeing that I could add anything to what she had already done. 'Of course,' she said yes, clutching at a straw.

Archie came into my clinic with Mum and Dad, plus siblings. They were a happy, noisy lot. Seeing them all together, I was struck by how very different Archie was to the rest of the family.

Yes, he had some facial features of his parents, but he was huge. When his growth was plotted on a growth chart, his height was in a similar range to that of his brother and sister, on the 75th centile, a little above average. But, while their weights were in the same range, his was so far above the 97th centile as to be almost off the chart!

I chatted with them.

'I guess he eats more than the rest of you?'

'Yes,' said Sylvia Thomas. 'He eats us out of house and home! We've tried so hard to help him cut it down, but he gets so distressed. We're at the end of our tether.'

I had a look at him. Apart from his vast size and a slightly elevated blood pressure, he was clinically well.

As I knew he was coming, I had done a little homework. One of my repeated moanings to students and trainees was 'No one ever reads the bloody literature!' I did my best to keep up, when I had a moment. I had discovered there was a relatively new hormone that had been discovered to control appetite: leptin. Low leptin levels made one eat a lot, but leptin levels rose when you had had enough to eat. It acted through a receptor in the brain. Naturally, I wondered whether this might be at the bottom of Archie's problem.

'I really don't know what's wrong with Archie, though I am absolutely certain that something is. I do not think for a moment that he is just greedy. There is just a possibility that he may have something wrong with a new hormone that has been discovered to affect appetite. There is a laboratory in London which can check the levels of this hormone, leptin. Shall we see whether they can help us?'

'Oh, yes,' they chorused. I said I would get back to them when I had set up a suitable investigation.

Later, I telephoned the professor who had been studying leptin. He was very excited.

'Arrange for him see my paediatric colleague and he will set up the relevant tests. Yes, it all sounds very promising!'

I heard nothing more for over a year. Then a paper was published, describing the first case in Britain of an abnormality of leptin production. This was Archie. The team had shown that he was making a non-functioning analogue of leptin, which meant that his appetite couldn't be suppressed; this was the reason he was eating so much.

In spite of our work on the putative identification of the Archie's problem, our team's contribution was not acknowledged.

Which brings me to Brian. Not long after this paper was published, I was at another regional paediatric meeting. The same paediatrician who had referred Archie to me came up.

'I've just heard about another boy, aged seven, who story is very like Archie's. He's a patient of Dr Bloomer's in Kent. She asked whether I knew anyone who could help and I suggested you.'

'Okay,' I said. 'I'll give her a ring.'

Brian duly appeared in my clinic. As I had been told, his story was almost exactly the same as Archie's. Nothing they had tried helped him to lose weight. I went through the same process and came to a similar conclusion.

'I think Brian may have an abnormality of leptin production'

I said, looking wise. 'I will arrange for Brian to have some special tests.' I referred him off to the same team.

A few weeks later I got a phone call from them, very excited. I was wrong about Brian. He made a normal copy of leptin, but the *receptor* for leptin that he made was abnormal and leptin couldn't bind to it.

In due course another paper was published. No mention of our team.

ANGELA

One anxiety that parents often have is whether their child is growing normally. It may be that they think he or she is too light, or that they are too short.

Children's growth charts are widely available and they suggest that increase in weight and height follow a smooth rise. Most parents will tell you that children don't grow like that and they are right.

For many years I taught that children grow in a series of steps. At one point, they wouldn't seem to grow much for a while, then they would suddenly start to eat more and then they would have a growth spurt, before slowing down again. I never tried to prove this; it was purely observational.

One day I attended a conference and an ex-SHO of mine came rushing up.

'Colin,' he said excitedly. 'I've just proved what you always said!'

'What was that?' I said, confused.

'About growth. I've just shown that children really do grow in spurts.'

He explained that he'd been carrying out a Medical Research Council funded project on children with genetic disorders, monitoring their growth. He had a group of healthy children as controls and was using a 'kneemometer' to measure their swinging leg length. This is a highly accurate method of following growth. He had found that children grow in a series of steps, as I had taught him. He also found that there was a bigger than usual increase in the Spring and a slightly smaller one in the Autumn. In between there were lesser spurts. This was very gratifying.

Madeleine Bright's question was rather different. She had three daughters, the youngest of whom, Angela, was fourteen. Deborah was the eldest at twenty, followed by Christine, who was eighteen. They were six foot two inches and six foot one inch respectively. She wanted to know how tall Angela was going to be and whether anything could be done to limit her final height.

'How do you feel about being tall?' I asked Angela.

'Oh, I'm not sure. Mother thinks it might be a nuisance, but Debs and Chrissie quite like being tall. They think it's cool to stand out a bit.'

'Do you want me to estimate how tall you're going to be? It means having an X-ray, which is ethically not really appropriate, unless you want to know.'

'Is there any other way?'

'Not to be as precise, but, if I measure you accurately myself over a period of three months, we can make a fairly good guess.'

'Let's do that, then.'

Angela and her mother came back and I measured her. There's a technique called 'mastoid distraction' that I used to employ, because it reduced the difference that posture can make on different occasions. You put your hands on the mastoid processes, just behind the ears, and push up. This straightens the spine a little and, although its reliability has been questioned, it makes measurements taken by the same person at different times easier to compare.

We met to decide what to do next.

'I think that Angela will end up around the same height as her sisters, between six foot one and six foot two. How do you feel about that, Angela?'

'It's cool.'

'Would you like to be less than six foot tall?'

'I think it might be better in the long run,' interjected Madeleine Bright. 'What would it entail?'

'Either giving Angela some medicine to accelerate the fusion of the ends of her long bone; her epiphyses; or surgery. I wouldn't be keen on either, frankly. There is good research to show that the hormone treatment works. However, psychological studies have shown that children who were dissatisfied with the prospect of being taller than average were just as dissatisfied after their final height had been reduced. So, it's not really much help.'

'I'm quite happy to be the same sort of height as my sisters,' said Angela.

At that, mother seemed to accept it.

'As long as you're happy,' she said.

OSWALD

There are a few principles about getting children who have had illnesses that impaired their growth to start growing again. Oswald was one of those.

He had been born in south London and failed to thrive from about nine months of age. It took quite a long time for his cœliac disease to be identified, by which time his weight was well below the third centile on the growth chart. He was put on a gluten-free diet and followed up locally by the community paediatric team and their dieticians.

After six months of his diet, Oswald still wasn't putting on weight. I had a phone call from one of the community paediatricians, asking me to see him.

Oswald and his mother, Prudence Edwards, met me in my clinic. He certainly was a scrawny little thing. Dr Michaels, one of the community doctors, came too.

'Since he started on his diet, he's been much happier,' said Mrs Edwards. 'He had these horrid nappies, but now his poos are small, but fairly well formed. He is quite good about eating his diet, but he just won't put on the weight he ought to. His length isn't increasing much either.'

I took a quick look at him. I had a lot of information about him already, from his multiple consultations. He was skinny and I couldn't feel his liver edge. He didn't have much subcutaneous fat.

'What does he eat each day?' I asked.

Prudence handed me his diet sheet. 'This is the plan we've been using. He does take it all.'

I looked at the sheet. All Oswald's foods were carefully listed.

As the dietician had drawn it up, she had given the calories provided by each of them. I looked at his total daily intake.

'He's not getting enough,' I declared.

'Yes, he is,' said Jenny Michaels. 'You can see he's getting plenty of calories for his weight.'

'Exactly,' I said. 'But he *isn't* getting enough calories for the weight he *ought* to be. He won't grow until he does.'

'Why not?' she asked.

'That's an interesting question,' I said. 'First of all, children who have lost weight don't grow, as a rule, unless you feed them enough for their expected weight. No one knows why, but I think the answer is probably quite simple. When they are ill, they don't put on weight, but their cells continue to divide. When they start treatment, their body cell numbers have increased, but the size of each cell is smaller than it should be. What I suspect we are having to do is to feed them according to the number of cells in their bodies, rather than their body mass.'

'That makes sense,' said Mrs Edwards.

'I suppose so,' said Dr Michaels grudgingly.

We increased Oswald's calorie intake to the right level. After a couple of weeks, he began to grow quite fast. Everyone was happy again.

9.

The Subtle Streptococcus

JULIAN

Julian was a thirteen-year-old boy who was referred to my clinic because of what were described as 'peculiar behaviours'. Dr Angel, his GP, said it had been first noticed at school. His teachers said that his attention seemed to be wandering and that he had become very fidgety. As he was a particularly bright boy, they had become concerned.

Mrs Maeve O'Connell, his mother, came with him to the outpatient appointment. She was a soft-faced lady with a ruddy complexion, dressed smartly for her hospital visit.

'We had noticed it too,' she said. 'He's been complaining of headaches, which isn't like him. He's dropped things without any obvious reason and, when I ask him something, he'll screw up his face. Sometimes he jerks his head or his shoulder. We thought it was a new habit.'

'Has he been unwell in the last year?'

'Only the usual: coughs, colds, the odd sore throat. He was off school about six months ago with a temperature and a cough. We thought he had 'flu.'

Julian was a healthy-looking boy. I went over to shake his hand.

'Mind if I have a look at you?'

'No,' he replied, standing up and holding out his hand. I shook it. His grip was unusual; he gripped my hand, then loosened his grip, then tightened again. Oh boy, I thought, 'milkmaid's grip'. That is rare, but so characteristic, we had a diagnosis.

Apart from mild hypotonia of all his limbs, his examination was normal.

'Has he been his usual self otherwise? Nothing out of the ordinary in his behaviour?'

'I'm okay,' Julian said. 'It's just a n.n.n.nuisance, is all.'

'Yes, he's developed a bit of a stammer too,' said Maeve.

'I think he has something called Sydenham's chorea,' I said. 'It's quite rare nowadays. It comes some months after having a throat infection with a Group A beta haemolytic streptococcus (GABHS) and is to do with his immune response to it. There are one or two other rare conditions that are like this, such as the PANDAS group of disorders (paediatric autoimmune neuropsychiatric disorders associated with streptococcal infection) and Gilles de la Tourette syndrome. His odd handshake, though, has only been described in Sydenham's chorea, so far as I know.'

'What can we do about it?'

'Two things. We need to do some tests to confirm the diagnosis and we need to put him on some treatment. Although the GABHS infection that started it off was quite a while ago, we want to make sure he doesn't get another one, so he needs to have regular treatment with penicillin. We can also try him on a drug called haloperidol. This may control his odd movements quite well, but the dose is critical, so he needs to come into the ward so that we can get his treatment exactly right.'

Julian came into the ward for ten days or so. His investigations showed that his antistreptolysin titre (ASOT) was very high, along with other markers of inflammation. Careful titration of haloperidol controlled his twitches, jerks and grimacing quite well.

About half of children with Sydenham's chorea recover over a few months. I weaned Julian off his haloperidol after he had been free of symptoms for about six months. None of his unusual behaviours returned.

ROSALIE

Rosalie was six years old. She was originally under the care of a colleague, but had only attended one appointment before my colleague went on holiday, so I met her instead.

She came with her mother, Alice Keyes. The family had returned recently from Washington, where David Keyes was a Junior Secretary in the British Embassy. The family were a branch of a family well established in English politics and diplomacy.

Rosalie's problems had begun in Washington. She developed a red blotchy rash, headaches and intermittent joint pains without inflammation, we'd call it arthralgia. Red, swollen lumps appeared on the palms of her hands and the soles of her feet, lasted a few days and then disappeared. These came and went at unpredictable intervals. She was, at times, rather lethargic and, early in the illness, had developed a low-grade fever, although this also subsided before the family returned to England, at the end of her father's tour of duty.

This mysterious illness had led to visits to several specialists in Washington. She had been seen by a local paediatrician, a professor of paediatric dermatology, another professor of paediatric endocrinology and, finally, a professor of paediatric neurology. They had carried out a multitude of investigations but had not confirmed a diagnosis. However, the dermatologist had started a course of oral steroid treatment which had suppressed her symptoms to some extent, but not abolished them.

I met them in my clinic initially; Rosalie was a very chatty, cheerful girl.

'You're the seventh doctor I've seen!' she remarked. 'Are you any good?'

'You'll have to tell me what you think later,' I said. 'That's for you to judge.'

'Okay,' she agreed.

Alice and I went through her copious notes. They had brought all the American results. One or two tests caught my eye.

'She had a raised ASOT, ESR and CRP early on,' I pointed out. 'What did the US doctors think of that?'

'They said it didn't mean much,' said Mrs Keyes. 'She doesn't fulfil the Jones criteria for rheumatic fever and they said it just meant she's had a strep infection in the past and had some inflammation.'

The Jones criteria, major and minor, have been used for years to make a diagnosis of rheumatic fever, though some would say that they aren't quite so useful today, because we understand the wider impact of GABHS infections now.

'Do you have any symptoms at the moment?' I asked Rosalie.

'Oh yes. Look,' she showed me her hands. There were some reddish lumps on her palms, between 5 and 10 mm in diameter.

'Do they hurt?'

'Only when I press them.'

'Anything else?'

'She's been having some headaches,' said her mother.

'Not now,' said Rosalie.

'What about your joints?'

'Yes, they ache sometimes. They're not too bad today.'

I examined Rosalie. Apart from the lumps on her hands and two on her feet, she had a blotchy rash on her lower legs and her tummy.

'Do these come and go?' I asked.

'Yes,' said Rosalie.

'Is Rosalie still on treatment?'

'I've been reducing her prednisolone slowly, since we came last,' said Alice Keyes. 'She's only having 2.5 milligrams every other day now.' Prednisolone was the steroid she was on. The dose was almost homeopathic.

'Well, let's go on reducing it and see what happens.'

By her next visit, Rosalie was off her treatment and they came to my office, rather than my clinic.

'How are you?' I asked.

'Fine!' said Rosalie, immediately turning to her mother and saying, 'Not fine!'

Alice Keyes and I laughed. In the lift, Mrs Keyes had said to Rosalie, 'Now, you must tell Dr Stern today that you haven't been quite so well.' When she came in and sat down, Rosalie gave the polite reply 'Fine!' and then realised she should have said 'Not fine!'

Her symptoms had all come back. We repeated her investigations. Her ASOT was again raised, as were her markers of inflammation. We started her back on her steroids, at a low dose and I added oral penicillin, as I suspected that this was another post GABHS disease, though it didn't quite fit the ones I knew about.

Later that month, I was asked to organise a regional paediatric clinical meeting. I thought it would be fun to ask my colleagues to present mystery cases, where no one had made a satisfactory diagnosis. We had a competition for the best presentation. One of my SHOs presented Rosalie's case. He was very good and won! We didn't manage to solve any of the cases, though.

A week later, I was doing my usual regular rummage through the literature. I came across a paper published five years before in an obscure journal, describing seven cases that had presented at a children's hospital over a period of twenty years. They were all identical to Rosalie's case. They were all thought to have a post GABHS illness. At last!

Rosalie took a year or two to settle down, but eventually all her symptoms faded away, helped by the steroid therapy. She stayed on oral penicillin.

I spent a year, actually two academic terms, teaching at the King Saud University in Riyadh. From a clinical point of view, this was fascinating. I remember speaking to another, Saudi, Professor, when I arrived, knowing that there was a 30 per cent cousin marriage rate.

'You must see lots of genetic disorders.'

'Not at all. The prevalence of cystic fibrosis here is similar to that in the United Kingdom.'

He was quite right. However, there **was** a great deal of inherited disease. I saw many conditions that were very rare in Britain and several that were unique to the Saudi Kingdom. This happened largely because I was given the responsibility of looking after the paediatric intensive care unit, where many of these children ended up.

However, one case that stuck out was really quite a common one.

AMIR

Amir Hassan was a ten-year-old boy whose Swedish mother, Gudrun Hassan, had found lying on the floor of their bathroom having a generalised epileptic fit. Gudrun was a gynaecologist at the university hospital, where I worked, so she brought him in to the Children's A&E.

The initial investigations found that he had high blood pressure and observations there suggested a renal origin. He was transferred to the renal team. For reasons I couldn't establish, they decided that he was lacking in fluid, so they set up an intravenous infusion, giving him quite large amounts of dextrose saline solution. His convulsions kept recurring. Being unable to control them, they transferred him to my care.

I was sitting at my desk looking at his medical notes, when I became aware that someone was looking over my shoulder. I looked round. It was, in my opinion, the less than competent professor of nephrology. I had shared an office with him briefly. He had upset me two days after I arrived, by telling me I should come with him to the main square.

'Why is that?' I asked.

'There's a beheading!' he said, somewhat gleefully. I politely declined to go.

'What are you doing?' he asked now, somewhat belligerently.

'Reading Amir's notes,' I said, neutrally.

'It's obvious, he's in status epilepticus.'

'Well, he was, but we have controlled his seizures now.'

'What's the cause?'

'When he came in, there was some blood in his urine, There still is, though he isn't passing much.'

'We know that!'

'He had a sore throat a few days ago. I think he has post-streptococcal glomerulonephritis.'

'Nonsense!' he said and stomped off.

Of course, that was exactly what he had. It follows soon after an infection with the GABHS. We cut down his fluids, managed him conservatively until his glomerulonephritis settled down and slowly, he recovered. It's a fairly common condition, but I will say more about it later.

His father, Mohammed Hassan, turned out to be the King's

Chief Justice. I think, had I run into any legal problems while I was there, he would have been an enormous help.

It's interesting that one type of bacterium can lead to such a variety of post-infectious patterns of disease. The popular and accepted theory is based on the idea of molecular mimicry. In this, the immune system, in responding to the GABHS infection, is supposed to find molecules in human tissues that are so similar that it makes a response to them, causing what's known as an autoimmune disease.

I have always found this a very unsatisfactory explanation, in spite of the repeated description in the literature of antibodies that interact with specific sites on human cells.

I doubt these explanations for two reasons. Firstly, it seems to me intrinsically unlikely that the immune system, which has developed sophisticated ways of identifying what is 'self' and what isn't, would be subverted so easily. Secondly, although there are a number of autoimmune diseases, for the majority, explanations as to how they arise are lacking.

In post GABHS disease, I suggest a much simpler mechanism. The streptococcus has a polysaccharide coat which carries a strongly positive electric charge. When the immune system destroys the bacterium, this coat is released, but cannot be easily digested by the body, so it circulates until it is excreted. If enough of the polysaccharide passes through the kidney, it will become trapped by the basement membrane of the glomerulus, which is the kidney's filter mechanism. This basement membrane has a strong negative electric charge, so the polysaccharide will bind tightly to it. The immune response to GABHS finds this polysaccharide antigen in the kidney and attacks it, leading, in this instance to post GABHS glomerulonephritis. The appearance of the affected kidney on microscopy fits this mechanism exactly. It would take some months for the polysaccharide to leach out of the kidney. This tallies well with the progress of the disease, which take about a year to fade away, judging by the persistence of blood in the urine.

I think that the other post GABHS diseases occur in analogous ways, because basement membranes carrying negative charges are found in a number of other places: the brainstem (chorea), joints (arthritis), the heart (rheumatic heart disease), skin (rheumatic-type rashes) and so on. Depending upon how much polysaccharide is circulating and its average molecular size may determine which tissue it binds to and which type of post GABHS develops.

10.

Looking and Listening

HENRY

Sometimes finding a diagnosis can be difficult, but often the keys to sorting out a tricky problem are either to listen to the story more carefully, then examine the patient more thoroughly, and not to discard the suggestions of another professional too quickly.

After completing work on my PhD, I was appointed as a Senior Lecturer in Immunology at the Royal Postgraduate Medical School, with an Honorary Consultancy in Paediatrics. There was an interval of a year before Professor John Humphrey was opening his department and I could take up the post, so I spent a year as a locum consultant in paediatrics at a district general hospital. I learnt a lot while I was there.

Henry was a baby of nine months of age who was brought to the A&E Department because he was vomiting frequently and not putting on weight. His condition was poor and the team admitted him under my care. I saw him with his parents, Angela and Sean Boughton.

'He was doing really well at first,' Angela Boughton said. 'He was easy to feed and settled really well. Then he seemed to get a bit anxious about feeding and to bring up a little bit more than he had been. Before that he only posseted a little. As time went by he vomited more and more. He seems to be worse in the mornings than later in the day. Recently, he is losing weight, whereas before it was just that he wasn't gaining as much as he should.'

I went over the history obtained by the doctors in training on my team. There wasn't a lot more to add.

'Is he still passing stools?'

'Only a little now, dirty nappies are becoming less frequent.'

Henry was a small, rather wizened baby. I thought he looked a bit dehydrated. He hadn't shown signs of a fever, or of any infection.

'Do we have his blood results?'

'Yes,' said Dr Ahmed, my Registrar. 'His serum sodium is on the low side and he's slightly alkalotic. He's a little anaemic, but his white cell count and CRP are normal.'

These results suggested that his vomiting was quite significant, backed up the idea that he was too dry and confirmed that infection was less likely.

'Let's set about putting up a drip with normal saline to begin with. We'll take it slowly,' I suggested.

While the team were sorting that out, I started to examine him. Near the end, I picked up an ophthalmoscope in order to examine his eyes. This is difficult in a baby, because they don't like having a bright light shone into their eyes, so one has to be patient and be fairly practiced at it. I spent a while doing this.

I was not happy with the appearance of the optic fundi. These are at the back of each eye, near the middle of the retinae, at the place where the optic nerve runs from the eye to the brain. Henry's fundi looked rather swollen to me, as though they were being pushed slightly into the eye. This condition, known as papilloedema, is unusual in babies under a year, as the skull bones haven't fused and can stretch a little to accommodate swelling of the brain. I tried to see whether Henry's fontanelle, the soft spot at the top of a baby's skull, was protruding, but it had closed too far for me to tell.

I turned to his parents. 'The first thing we need to do is to make sure that his general condition is improved. He is a bit dry and his blood chemistry needs to be put right. We'll give him some fluids into a vein and that should do the trick.'

They nodded their understanding. 'Why do you think he is vomiting?' asked Mrs Boughton.

'I think that it's due to increased pressure inside his skull,' I replied. 'The easiest way to find out what's going on is to carry out a CT scan of his head, as well as some other imaging studies.' Henry's illness was long before these tests were available widely. 'We'll need to transfer him to a children's hospital where they can do all these tests.'

'Can we go with him?'

'Of course. I will go and make the arrangements now.'

Henry's parents hadn't asked me what the exact cause might be. I was fairly sure that he had a brain tumour, possibly a medulloblastoma, and that it was imperative that he went to a paediatric neurosurgical unit as soon as possible.

In this hospital we didn't have the equipment, or the appropriate staff, to carry out imaging studies on the brain of an infant. Furthermore, although possibly a lumbar puncture might have been indicated by the physical signs, in his case it could be dangerous. Doing so might allow his brainstem to slip down into the top of his vertebral canal, a process known as 'coning', which is often fatal.

I went to my office and spoke to one of the neurosurgical team at the children's hospital on the phone. They had a cot available and we arranged to transfer him that day. I breathed a sigh of relief. At least we had done what we could and I hoped that he would be lucky, although the outcome for brain tumours in infants of this age was very poor in those days and hasn't improved all that much today.

I expected to have some feedback about him, but we heard nothing. I had almost forgotten about the case when I had a phone call in my clinic six weeks later.

'Can you spare a minute?' said Dr Ahmed. 'I think you need to see this little boy urgently.'

I made my apologies to the clinic sister and said I would be back shortly. A&E was nearby. When I arrived, the patient was Henry.

He was in a worse state that when I first saw him. There was no sign that he had been operated on. His mother looked at me tearfully.

'What happened at GOS?' I asked.

'They said they couldn't find anything wrong with him,' she replied. 'A doctor came and examined him, said he was fine and to take him home. He was only there for a day.'

I re-examined Henry. The papilloedema was more pronounced than ever, which wasn't a surprise.

'I think they are wrong,' I said. 'We must send him back straight away. Last time I spoke to a more junior member of their team. This time I will speak to the Professor.'

I went to my office and, after being sent round the houses a few times, eventually got him on the phone. He was as shocked as I, having never even being told about Henry's previous admission. He took him back immediately and we sent the Boughtons off in another ambulance.

A few days later, the neurosurgical Professor telephoned me to tell me that poor little Henry had died.

'His medulloblastoma was too advanced for me to be able to do anything. Actually, given his history, had I seen him six weeks earlier, it's unlikely we could have helped him then, but you never know.'

It eventually emerged that Henry had been examined on his first admission by the team's Senior Registrar, who was a rather overbearing individual. He had disregarded my clinical opinion and overruled it. He was censured by his boss.

I discussed the case with my team. 'Never ignore the opinions of others,' I said. 'They may have spotted something you've missed. In fact, mother is always right! She may not know *why* something is happening, but her observations are crucial in solving her child's problems.'

JEAN

Jean Bateman lived near Southampton. She was fifteen years old and had been referred to me by her family doctor, who had been a student at my hospital. She arrived with her mother,

Melanie. They were both dressed very smartly, obviously planning to enjoy a day up in London, after coming to see me.

Her problem was fatigue. For the previous two years, Jean had found it more and more difficult to manage her life. In particular, getting up and going to school took a lot out of her. When she came home, she needed to rest on her bed for an hour or two and, to save time, would try to get through any homework she had while eating her supper.

This was in contrast to her way of life before. She was a high achiever and had been in several school and local sports teams. While she was managing to hold her own academically, she had been compelled to give up her sports for the time being. She was complaining sometimes of joint pains, occasional headaches and skin rashes that came and went.

Having learned all this from her referral letter, I was about to start taking a history, when Jean asked whether she could speak to me on her own. I was rather reluctant, because of the issue of her having a chaperone.

'All right,' I said, compromising. 'We can have a chat together while your mother waits outside. Then she'll have to come in again, when it's time for me to have a proper look at you. Would that be acceptable?' Mother and daughter agreed. We stood up as Mrs Bateman left the room.

Jean and I sat down. 'When did all your problems start?'

'About two years ago. We'd just come back from holiday and I was about to go back to school. Then I got a skin rash on my leg and pains in my joints. I took some Panadol and it got a bit better. I went back to school, but, after a week or two, I began to feel more and more tired. My headaches started, and the rashes and joint pains came and went. Ever since then it just got worse. My friends think I'm faking it all, but I'm not!' She became tearful. This was why she didn't want her mother there, I thought.

'I'm sure we can find out what's going wrong,' I said, reassuringly. 'Tell me, where had you been on holiday?'

'America.'

'That must have been fun,' I said.

'It was,' Jean replied. 'We go regularly,' she amplified. 'My aunt and uncle and my cousins live there, so we stay with them. We always have a good time.'

'Whereabouts do they live?' I asked.

'In Connecticut, in New England. They have a lovely house in the country. There's a lake and a boat and lots to do.'

'Do you go for walks?' I asked.

'Every day. It's a bit of a ritual. Once a day, often after breakfast, but sometimes after supper, depending upon what we do, we take a walk all together in the woods. There's a gate at the bottom of their garden – they call it a yard – that goes straight into the forest, if we turn right. Turning left takes us to the lake.'

'That's all I need to know.' I said. Let's get your mother back in now.' Jean looked a bit surprised.

'Is that all?' Jean asked.

'Well, I think I know what your problem is now and I think your mother should be here when I go through it.'

'Oh, okay.'

Mrs Bateman returned and sat down.

'I am fairly sure that your daughter has Lyme Disease,' I said.

To my surprise, Melanie Bateman clapped her hand to her head, said, 'I'm so cross!' and burst into tears.

'Don't worry, we can do a blood test to check it out and then put Jean on the right antibiotic combination. There's a good chance that she'll be entirely back to normal soon.'

'I know,' she said. 'It's not that she can't be made better. I'm so cross that I didn't think of it.'

'Why on earth should you?' I asked.

At that time, Lyme Disease was uncommon in the United Kingdom. Only a handful of cases had been described, all in the New Forest area, but it was much more common in New England. It's caused by a particular bacterium, Borrelia burgdorferi, and carried by the deer tick. If an infected tick bites someone, it can infect them with the bug.

'Everyone knows about Lyme Disease in Connecticut. When we go on walks with my sister's family, she always makes sure that her boys tuck their trouser bottoms into their socks, to reduce the risk of being bitten. I ought to have thought of it!'

'Never mind,' I said, slightly at a loss. 'We'll get on with Jean's tests after I have checked her out and I will take a chance and write up her treatment now. Once she has had the bloods taken, she can start it as soon as you get home.'

Jean's blood tests confirmed the diagnosis and she made a full recovery.

TIMOTHY

Sometimes, the problems a child may complain about can be hard to pin down. After all, patients, adult or child, rarely come to say, 'I've got pneumonia', or 'I have appendicitis'. They have headaches, or tummy ache or feel giddy. That was the case with Timothy, or Tim as he preferred to be called.

Tim's referral letter told me that this fourteen-year-old boy had been complaining of headache and episodes of dizziness for four years. These symptoms interfered with his schoolwork and his sports. His parents, Jeremy and Stella Wright, had sought opinions from a number of specialists: their local paediatrician in Essex, a neurologist, a psychiatrist and a Professor of paediatric neurology. They came to me when I was a Senior Lecturer in Immunology and also an Honorary Consultant in Paediatrics.

I took a careful history. His symptoms had started when he was ten. They were occasional to start with, becoming more frequent and disabling as time passed. Their vagueness had prompted suggestions that he was imagining them, or making them up, but this didn't fit with his personality, not did there seem to be any reason that he should malinger. My principle has always been to believe what I am told. By this time, everyone was sure that his problems were genuine, but couldn't find a cause.

'Where are your headaches?' I asked.

'Usually on top of my head, sometimes at the sides.'

'Both sides of your head equally?'

'Usually, though I sometimes think they are a bit worse on the left side.'

'What is the dizziness like? Does the room go round, or from side to side? If it goes round, which was does it go?'

'No, it seems as though my head is swimming about; more sideways.'

'Does it make you feel sick?'

'Sometimes.'

'Do you have the headaches and the dizziness at the same time?'

'Sometimes,' Tim repeated.

None of this was particularly illuminating. I continued to probe at the story without turning up anything very helpful. I thought I ought to move onto the clinical examination. This had always been entirely normal, when others had carried it out. In particular, detailed and careful neurological examinations had been normal. Interestingly, although he'd had some blood tests, which had all been fine, Tim hadn't had any imaging studies carried out.

Like everyone else had reported, everything was normal. I always look into the ears, strictly speaking the external auditory canals, the first time that I see most children. I did so here.

While peering in carefully, his left canal looked a bit odd. There was some wax in it, but, embedded in the wax there seemed to be something pink. This was not the pink of healthy human tissue, rather the colour of something artificial, like plastic.

'Have you stuck anything into your ear?' I asked Tim.

'No!' he replied.

'Well,' I said, 'There seems to be something in there that

shouldn't be there. I will get one of my ENT (Ear Nose and Throat) colleagues to have a look and, if possible, pull it out.'

'Will that take long?' asked Stella Wright.

'Let's see. I'll give him a ring.'

I paged one of the ENT Senior Registrars, as there was one on call for urgent consultations. As it happened, it was quiet that morning.

'Send him round to A&E,' he said. 'I'll see what I can do.'

'Send him back when you've finished with him,' I said. 'I will still be in clinic.'

The Wrights went off to A&E with a note from me. I asked them to come back when whatever it was had been removed.

They duly returned about an hour later. Tim was clutching a plastic pot, which he handed to me. It contained a Chinese chequer.

'We wondered where that had gone!' said Jeremy Wright. 'It disappeared about four years ago. The whole family were playing Chinese Chequers and one went missing. We though it must have rolled under a skirting board.'

'This must have been about the same time you developed your symptoms,' I said to Tim.

'I suppose so.'

'Well, I don't know whether it has anything to do with them, but let's wait and see.'

I followed him up for three months or so. None of Tim's funny turns ever came back. After the Chinese chequer was removed, he was as right as rain.

I can't say definitely that having the chequer stuck in his ear was the cause of Tim's headaches and dizziness. However, it seems probable, because the nerve that supplies that part of the body, when stimulated, can cause symptoms of that sort.

The moral of this story is that, whatever preconceptions you may have about a case, it pays always to carry out a thorough physical examination. It seems possible that, before he came to see me, no one had looked into Tim's ears.

PHILIP

While working as an Honorary Senior Registrar, another fourteen-year-old boy presented with a very unusual problem.

Philip French had been suffering from a rash that recurred every three weeks for a period of eighteen months. He would feel a little unwell just before the rash appeared with a low-grade fever. As the rash came out, his fever would subside. The spots were primarily on his legs, especially behind his knees, and also on his upper arms and buttocks. They faded over a period of ten days or so, only to reappear at this remarkably regular interval.

He was admitted during one of the episodes through our A&E Department and I met him with his mother, Edna French, on my ward round. His history had been taken meticulously by our team and he had been thoroughly examined. Apart from his skin rash, nothing was found in particular. His investigations showed that his ESR and CRP were a little elevated; these are non-specific signs of inflammation and so in keeping with his condition. All his other routine tests were normal, apart from a trace of blood in his urine.

I discussed the situation with Mrs French.

'If it weren't for the recurrent nature of his rash, I would have thought that Philip was suffering from a condition called Henoch-Schönlein purpura. We don't know what causes this condition, but it is benign and, in all the other cases I have seen, subsides over two or three weeks. Obviously, that isn't what is going on here.'

'What is it then?' Edna French asked.

'There are some rare cases of recurrent Henoch-Schönlein purpura and it seems probable that this is what Philip has. Again, we don't know why this happens. However, it most probably is the result of something not quite right in his immune system. I'm also working in the Department of Immunology, so I will discuss Philip with my colleagues there and we'll think about what we might be able to do to help. May he stay with us for a day or two?'

'Of course, if you think it would help,' she agreed.

As he had a few more red blood cells in his urine than we would normally expect to find, we followed up that lead. There are always some red cells in the urine, but nothing special came of that, other than that the rate of excretion of red blood cells in his urine was higher than normal.

I discussed Philip's case with my immunological colleagues. My boss, the Professor of Immunology, spoke up.

'One thing you could do is ask June to have a look at his plasma.'

June was a consultant in virology and a world authority on the electron microscopy of viruses. I went to have a word with her.

'Okay,' she said. 'Get me a blood sample, I'll spin it down and have a look.'

I did so. Two days later June gave me a call.

'That blood sample you sent me,' she began. 'I had a look at the plasma and it's quite interesting. Come and have a look.'

This was a comment of great excitement from June, a devotee of litotes.

We look at the photomicrographs she had taken. She pointed out something that looked to me like an amorphous blob.

'I'm sure that's a mycoplasma,' she said. 'His plasma sample is full of them. I haven't seen them before in a specimen like this.'

This was a fascinating lead. The mycoplasma family are a group of organisms that are neither bacteria not viruses, but somewhere in between. Some types are known to cause illnesses in humans, such as pneumonia, but they had never been implicated in Henoch-Schönlein purpura.

I went away to follow this up. We sent off blood samples to look for antibodies against mycoplasma, but they came back negative. This didn't put me off, because these tests are very type-specific and it could easily be a new variety.

I wondered what else we could do. Then I remembered the trace of blood in his urine. We had a team meeting.

'Mycoplasma are quite sensitive to antibiotics of the erythromycin family, the macrolides. I suggest we make a timed collection of urine and calculate Philip's red cell urinary excretion rate. Then we can start him on a prolonged course of clarithromycin and check his red cell urinary excretion rate every alternate day.'

We started Philip on clarithromycin. Within four days, the excretion of red cells in his urine dropped to normal. We continued his antibiotic for twelve weeks. No further episodes of his skin rash returned, so I stopped his treatment. Some eight weeks later, the rashes came back again and red cell numbers rose in his urine.

'All right,' I said to Philip and his mother. 'We need to continue his treatment indefinitely for the moment.'

'Why has the rash come back?' asked Philip.

'To be honest, we don't know, but I can speculate. I think that this particular mycoplasma is hiding in your liver, probably in what we call the venous sinusoids. You must have antibodies to it in your blood stream that keep it under control most of the time, but there is likely to be a very minor abnormality in your immune system, especially against this bug, that means you never completely eliminate it. When the colonies of mycoplasma in your liver reach a critical size, they spill out into your blood stream. This starts off the rashes and also makes your kidneys bleed a little, a consequence of what we call an immune complex disease. After a while, the numbers of mycoplasma fall, being neutralised by your antibodies, but a few are left in the liver. Then the whole cycle starts again.'

'Will I never be rid of it?' Philip asked plaintively.

'I hope that you will, but, in the meantime, let's start your treatment again.'

We did that and, for the remainder of my time there, Philip stayed on treatment and was well.

I am sure that *all* cases of Henoch-Schönlein purpura are

caused by this unusual species of mycoplasma and, in a few rare instances such as Philip's, the disease becomes recurrent, because either of a minor immunological deficit, or, more likely, because of an underlying specific genetic background. No one agrees with me, so far as I'm aware, but no one has any other explanation.

MARIGOLD

While writing up my PhD thesis, I spent a year working as a locum consultant in paediatrics. Five-year-old Marigold came to my clinic because she was losing patches of hair. This had been a problem for several weeks, her mother, Suzie Smith, told me.

'A little bit more comes out whenever I brush her hair,' she said. 'It's leaving small circular holes.'

I had a quick look, using a small lens and a light. I could see the stumpy ends of hairs of irregular length, set in three round patches of baldness, each no more than 3 or 4 cm across.

'Marigold has a fungus infection of her scalp, called Tinea capitis. It's easy to treat; I'll give her some treatment for it.'

I took a scraping of her scalp to send to the laboratory, just to confirm my diagnosis.

'Here's a prescription for some anti-fungal cream. Put it on her scalp three times a day and she must continue it for six weeks, because the fungus grows slowly and so takes a long time to eliminate. If there's a problem and it doesn't go away, come back in a couple of months, otherwise, provided it does disappear, I don't need to see her again.'

Marigold and her mother left the clinic. I didn't expect to see her again, but, just over two months later, back they came.

'Oh dear,' I said. 'Didn't your hair grow back, then?'

'Oh yes,' said Suzie Smith. 'Have a look.'

I did and could see that her scalp had healed beautifully. 'What's the problem, then?'

'It's Granddad,' she replied. 'I wondered whether you'd see him too?'

'I'm a paediatrician,' I said. 'I don't treat grown-ups.'

She ignored me, went to the door and asked him to come in. He was a short, slightly overweight bald man in his late fifties.

'My parents live next door,' she continued. 'Grandma collects Marigold from school and she stays with them until I get home from work. As soon as they get home, Marigold runs up to Granddad, who is sitting by the fire, jumps onto his lap and they have a cuddle. A couple of weeks ago he said to me, 'Have a look at my scalp'. To my amazement, his hair had started to grow just above his right ear. We puzzled over this, as Dad's been bald since he was in his twenties! Then we realised that the hair had grown exactly where Marigold had been rubbing her head on his. We wondered whether the anti-fungal cream was to blame.'

I had a look at his head. True enough, normal hair was growing in a small patch over his left ear, but nowhere else. The rest of his scalp was smooth and bald, there were no signs of crusting or flaking, which one sometimes sees with fungal scalp infection. I decide to take a scraping anyway.

'What an interesting story,' I said. 'I can't see any evidence that your scalp is infected,' I said to Granddad. 'I'll send this off to the lab. In the meantime, I'll prescribe some of the cream for you to try out. You'll need to continue it for some time, I should think, should it prove helpful. I'll ask your GP to follow it up.'

Off they trooped. When the lab result came back, there was no sign of infection. I wrote to his doctor, telling him what had happened and asking him to continue the treatment, if it seemed to help.

I heard nothing. Then, about four months later, I arrived at my clinic to see Granddad sitting there. By now, he had a couple of centimetres of hair growing all over his head.

'It's worked!' he said, enthusiastically. He was delighted.

I have no idea whether it was coincidence or the cream that restored his head of hair. Sometimes you never know why.

11.

When Children are Victims

ANGELA

Child abuse can lead to non-accidental injury and it isn't always easy to be certain about the cause of these injuries. In Angela's case, I was asked to see her because her mother, Lesley Venables, was worried that she couldn't settle her at night.

Her GP couldn't find any reason for this, but Lesley was becoming increasingly anxious about this problem, so I was asked to have a look at her.

Angela was eighteen months old. Lesley said that, every time she put her down for a sleep, she would cry and nothing seemed to calm her down. During the day, she was all right and played happily. Ms Venables was working during the day, but said that her childminder was happy with her.

'Does she manage to sleep all right when she is there?'

'I think so. Alice (the childminder) hasn't complained. She says Angela's as good as gold when she's there. I don't know what the matter can be!' Lesley was obviously very upset.

I took a full birth and past history and they were all quite normal. Her growth was normal for her age and she was eating a healthy mixed diet. There was nothing in the family history to suggest a genetic disorder.

I examined Angela, who lived up to her name during the process. She was quite healthy and there were no signs of disease or injury.

Sometimes, in these circumstances, you get a feeling that you haven't been told what lies behind Mum's anxiety. I thought that might be the problem here.

'Angela is fine. Now tell me what you're really worried about.'

Lesley burst into tears. I gave her a box of tissues and let her cry for a bit. Then she pulled herself together.

'It's Brian,' she said. 'He's coming out next week.' More tears.

'Who is Brian?'

'He's my ex-partner and Angela's dad. He's threatened to kill me when he gets out.'

'Why?'

'Because I shopped him. He was knocking me about and I called the police. He got put away for two years, so Angela doesn't know him and I don't want her to.'

'Don't you have a protection order out against him?'

'No.'

'Why not?'

'I can't get social services to listen. They just put the phone down on my brother whenever he phones them up! He's been helping me.'

This was a very strange state of affairs, I thought. Brian shouldn't be allowed anywhere near Lesley and Angela, not only because of his history of violence against Lesley, but also because of his threats.

'Do you have regular visits from a social worker?'

'I used to, but they said I was doing so well, they didn't need to come any more.'

'Who was the last social worker you saw?'

'Catherine Potter. She was very nice, but I think she's moved now.'

I found out which team had been responsible for her care and phoned them up immediately. I spoke with the team manager.

It emerged that Lesley's family were well known to social services. Both Lesley parents, Tom and Ellie, had learning needs, as did both Lesley's brothers. Lesley herself was less badly affected and had coped at a normal school. The whole family had been receiving years of social support and, as a consequence, would phone up wanting help with the most minor issues.

This had led to a situation that, whenever a member of the family telephoned for help, social workers had developed a habit of hanging up on them. Unfortunately, one of Lesley's brothers had taken up the responsibility of getting help for Lesley and had been doing the telephoning. As he was known to have learning difficulties, no one listened properly to him!

I had a long talk with the team manager, who was horrified at the state of affairs. Between us, we obtained an emergency protection order for Lesley and Angela. It was arranged that Brian would be found accommodation a long way away from them.

After this, Angela slept well and so did Lesley.

STEPHEN

Stephen was a ten-year old boy who had a history of minor accidents. In the past, he'd broken his arm falling down the stairs, he'd fractured his wrist falling over playing football in the park, he'd suffered several sprains and bruises from time to time. All of these mishaps had been put down to his being a very active young boy, popular with his mates and who got up to a few pranks from time to time.

After the most recent accident, slipping off a skateboard at speed and getting a greenstick fracture of his fibula (a bone in the lower leg), the GP wondered whether he might have brittle bone disease, the common name for osteogenesis imperfecta. This history didn't seem quite right for that, because of the bruises and sprains, but he might have a condition that made his tendons and ligaments stretchier and weaker.

Steve arrived with his mother, Mrs Perks. She was a large and cheerful lady with a florid complexion. She brought a four-year-old daughter along, Lucy, who played with the toys. Steve, it emerged, was the oldest of six children: the others were at school, two girls aged six and seven, and two boys aged eight and nine. Mrs and Mrs Perks were starting to slow up!

'So, Steve seems to keep hurting himself.'

'Ooh yes, he's such an active boy. Can't keep him in one place. Always rushing about here, there and everywhere, into everything. Full of beans, he is.'

'Are you a bit clumsy, then Steve?'

'Dunno,' was the terse reply.

'It sounds as though you just lose your balance sometimes

and fall badly. Is that right?'

'Suppose so.'

I was getting nowhere fast.

'How about your friends, do they hurt themselves too?'

'Alfie fell off a wall once.'

'Did he break anything?'

'Naah, just got a big bruise.'

'Anyone else break anything?'

'Dunno.'

'Mind if I have a look at you?'

'Suppose so.' Not a large vocabulary here.

I examined Steve. Physically, he was healthy and I couldn't find any of the clinical signs that go with brittle bone disease, such a blueness of the sclera – the white if the eye. There was no sign that his limbs were capable of unusual hyperextension, suggesting his ligaments were normal.

He did, true to form, have some bruises.

'Where'd you get these?' I asked.

'Here and there.'

There were circular bruises around his upper arms.

'These too?'

'I suppose.'

He had a bruise on his left cheek with some linear striation.

'How about that?'

'Suppose.'

I was not at all happy. The bruises on his upper arms were typical of his having been held very tightly there, probably by an adult. The one on his cheek was also typical of a smack with the open palm of an adult right hand. I asked the clinic nurse to step in for a moment.

'Mrs Perks, please may we have a little chat on our own? The children can play here until we come back.'

Reluctantly, she agreed. Once on our own, I was able to be frank, without making it difficult for Steve, who was trying not to give the game away.

'The bruises on Steve's arms and the one on his cheek were definitely caused by someone, first holding him very tightly and then smacking him on his face. Do you know who did that?'

'Oh dear, he's a very good dad really, but he does drink too much. Stevie loves him, his dad doesn't mean it, but he can't help himself. It's the pub.' There we had it.

'Does Mr Perks go to the pub every night?'

'Of course, he has to. It's our pub!'

Mr and Mrs Perks both turned out to be alcoholics. Being publicans was definitely the wrong profession for them. Mrs Perks wasn't ever violent, but, when Mr Perks was violent, she was too drunk to stop him. Steve turned out to be the whipping boy for the family, the other children were never hurt.

This was quite a difficult one to sort out. Financially, they couldn't give up the pub. Legally, we had to protect the children. The local authority called for a Child Protection Conference. I made sure that I was present, along with the consultant who ran the drug and alcohol dependency unit. After lots of discussion and more than one meeting, we came to an agreement. Mr and Mrs Perks started treatment for their alcoholism. They were given a drug, disulfiram, that makes you vomit if you drink alcohol. Social services arranged regular supervision and checked out the children regularly.

Fortunately, all this effort paid off. The Perks stayed off the sauce and loyal Steve had no more 'accidents'.

OLIVER

One Monday morning on my ward round, we stopped beside a cot. Oliver, a baby of nine months, was lying in it, looking up at us and smiling.

'Tell me about Oliver,' I asked the SHO.

'He came in late last night, through Children's A&E,' Dr Peters said. 'His mother brought him in. She came back from an evening with friends and her babysitter said that Oliver had tried to climb out of his cot on the wrong side and slipped down between the cot and the wall. He lifted him out and found that, in his struggle to get free, he had developed some minor bruising. The A&E team checked him over, couldn't find anything else wrong with him and asked us to admit him for observation overnight.

'I looked at him when he came in. He seems happy and well. He had some bruising on the sides of his upper arms and on his legs and some small ones on his back. Otherwise he's okay.'

'Where is his mother?'

'Tracey Ellis? She's an eighteen-year-old single mum and she works in a shop. She was here earlier, but she's had to go to work. She doesn't have any other children.'

'When you spoke with her, did you think the story stacked up?'

'I think so. She was out with some of her girlfriends and this happened while she was out.'

'Did you ask about the babysitter?'

'Yes, he's Michael – I didn't get his other name. He's a friend of Tracey's and did it to help Tracey have an evening out.'

I took off Oliver's babygro and had a look at him. The bruises were as Nadia Peters described them. I looked at his legs. After a minute or two I turned to Nadia.

'What do you make of that?' pointing at Oliver's left leg, on one side of his upper calf.

'It's a sort of circular bruise.'

'Anything else?'

'The margins are a bit irregular.'

'What do you think made it?'

'I'm not sure.'

I let her out of her confusion. 'It's a bite mark. Here, you can see the irregularities and indentations made by teeth, both from the upper and lower jaws. What's more, from the size of it, the bite was from an adult, certainly within the last twelve hours or so. What now?'

'It has to be a case of non-accidental injury, doesn't it? We need to ask for an urgent case conference to decide on the next steps.'

'Absolutely. I need to speak with mother after she finishes work and she needs to meet social services. Is she known to them?'

'I don't know, I'll find out.'

We continued the ward round. Later, I met Tracey. I showed

her the bite mark. She was horrified.

'I don't know how he could have got that!' she said. 'There's been no one near him except me and I'd never do that.'

'What about Michael, your babysitter? By the way, what's his other name?'

'Michael Peacock. Oh, he's lovely, it couldn't have been him, I'm sure. He's babysat for all my friends and they've had no trouble.'

'Well, we need to find out how it happened and what we can do to keep Oliver safe. We'll set up a meeting with social services and the other important groups.'

'Oh, Sally Hancock knows me, she's my social worker.' This was the first indication that Tracey was 'known' to social services.

In due course Oliver's Child Protection meeting took place. Sally Hancock and I were there and another social worker, plus two police officers from their Child Protection team. It is statutory policy that the police are invited.

Most of the discussion centred around Tracey.

'We've known Tracey for a long time. She had a difficult childhood, got into bad company, was taking drugs and was in care for a while. But she's done really well. Of course, she didn't mean to fall pregnant, but we helped through it and she's been really good with Oliver; we have been so pleased with her.'

There was a lot of praise for her. I cut in.

'Yes, but what about Michael, the babysitter? Isn't he the most likely agent?'

'Well,' said Sally, 'We don't know a lot about him. He is

Tracey's new boyfriend, but they all say how nice he is.'

'We've had the forensic odontologist look at the bite and he thinks it was caused by a male adult. Michael has so far not given us a bite sample to check.'

One police officer leaned forward. He took out a photograph and showed it to everyone.

'Is this Michael?'

'Yes,' they all said.

'It's not our practice to contribute to these meetings, we're really just here to observe. However, we do have some relevant information to give you, which will, I think help. Michael Peacock is known to us. He was discharged from prison five months ago, after serving a two-year sentence for child abuse, including sexual abuse. I didn't tell you this, you understand.'

Nowadays, the protocols governing these meetings have become more inclusive, so information from almost any source may be heard.

Naturally, that put an entirely new focus on the case. Eventually, we were able to prove that Michael had bitten Oliver. In court, it was agreed that he was responsible for the injuries and he received a five-year sentence.

Tracey was mortified and vowed to take more care of Oliver in the future. I hope she managed to.

I have always believed in the importance of a patient's history and of maternal observations. I was once asked to speak at the annual meeting of the alumni of my medical school. As I was working in the associated teaching hospital, I suppose I was a convenient guest speaker. I forget the topic, but I know that I included with a quotation from a Victorian physician:

'Not enough attention is paid to the history of a patient.'

I said, foolishly, that it was the most useful and important thing in assessing a case. Taking questions afterwards, a grey-haired doctor at the back raised his hand.

'That's not what you taught me as a student,' he said, combatively. Help, I thought, I can't be that old!

'You told us that the most important thing to remember is that Mother Is Always Right!'

'True,' I admitted, 'It is the most important thing. I stand corrected.'

He was right, in both senses. But there are occasions when one has to realise that parents do get things wrong, sometimes. Most often, this is through no fault of their own.

ALAN

I met Alan on my ward round. He was three months old and had been brought to our Children's A&E by his grandmother.

'I had to bring him in,' she confessed. 'I didn't know what to do. He seems to be bringing everything up. His Mum, Angela, can't cope with him. I've been trying to help her out, but it's getting beyond me.'

'What's the problem with Angela?'

'Well, she's not doing anything, really. She sits in the living room watching the TV and Alan is in his cot. I got worried yesterday, so I went in and fed him. He seemed so hungry, poor little mite. And his clothes and nappy were filthy and wet.'

'Is Angela ill? Has she seen the doctor?'

'No, but I think she should. She hasn't been normal since Alan was born. I know it's difficult, being a single mum. I was, myself. But ever since she's been home with Alan, she doesn't seem to be interested.'

This sounded like a case of post-natal depression, to me. Strange, though, because I would have expected this to have been picked up, if not immediately after delivery, then on the community post-natal visits.

'Hasn't she been seen by the community midwife?'

'I don't think so.'

'Why not?'

'Well it may be because her delivery was a bit complicated. She was visiting her granny, my husband's mum, in Nottingham when she went into labour. She probably gave her address, but as soon as she came out of the maternity unit, she came back to London, to a new flat. Her granny has dementia, so she may not have been able to let the team up there know where she'd gone.'

It sounded like a perfect storm.

I looked at Alan. He had a slightly anxious look about him, probably wondering where his next meal was coming from.

I turned to Dr Ellis, the SHO.

'Did you find anything amiss?'

'He's rather undernourished, I think. He has some unusual marks on his bottom.'

I took off his nappy to have a look There were three or four reddish-purple patches close to his sacrum.

'What do you think these are?' I asked.

'I'm not sure. I've never seen anything quite like them.'

'To be honest, neither have I, but I think they are early bedsores!'

Babies are active creatures, so the likelihood of bedsores developing is very small. It emerged that Alan had been left lying in unchanged nappies for days at a time. He wasn't smiling when he came in, probably because he'd had virtually no interaction with Angela, or anyone else, for that matter. He'd been lying on his back, looking at the ceiling. No wonder he wasn't smiling and had bedsores.

We arranged for Angela to have treatment in a mother and baby unit for her severe post-natal depression. Once we had healed Alan's skin, fed him properly and got him smiling and gurgling, he joined her there. I was told that, after being given proper community support, there were no more serious problems.

As with Alan, neglect can follow when care given by healthy parents with significant learning difficulties isn't picked up and the right help provided.

SIMON AND EFFIE

I was on my ward round once when two children, Simon aged two and his sister, Effie, aged four, were admitted to the ward. They were severely underweight. We discovered that their parents, George and Delilah, were both known to have learning problems but, like Alan's mum Angela, had moved recently and were unsupported.

The children were starving because George and Delilah hadn't been giving them enough to eat, not from malignant intent, but because they simply weren't able to care for them adequately.

We gave George and Delilah something for tea. I was about to offer George a second banana but, when I turned round with it, I found him trying to eat the skin of the first one! He was so hungry.

Again, once a suitable network of support was established, George and Delilah thrived.

SUSAN

A similar problem arose when I was spending a year as a locum consultant, while writing up my PhD thesis.

Eliza and John were a couple with learning difficulties who met at a support group. Eliza had already given birth to two children, but it was decided that she wasn't able to look after them, so they were taken into care.

Eliza and John set up home together and, after a while, Susan was born. Local social services did their best to support them, but didn't think they were managing very well. I was asked to bring Susan into my ward for closer observation, to see how her parents were managing.

I met them on my ward round. Eliza was a soft-faced redhead, who was cradling Susan. John was a gentle, quiet man.

'Hello,' I said, 'How are you and how's Susan?'

'She's okay,' said Eliza.

'Have you any problems with her?'

'No,' said John.

'How often do you feed her?' I asked Eliza.

'When she needs it,' said Eliza.

'When's that?'

'Well, she cries.'

'How many times does she feed every day?'

'I'm not sure.'

'How often do you think she should be fed?'

'When she wants.'

'How often does she have a dirty nappy?'

'I'm not sure.'

Obviously, I wasn't getting very far. I examined Susan. She was a little underweight, but otherwise a healthy baby girl.

'Let's see how we get on over the rest of the week,' I said to the ward sister, Nancy Cummins. 'We'll help Eliza develop a regime for Susan and make sure there's a plan for her care that can be used at home.'

Everything went well and Eliza managed to get the hang of how to care for Susan. With enough support at home, I thought, they would be all right.

The social work team manager telephoned to see how things were going.

'How often were your staff visiting them before she came in?' I asked.

'Once a week, but, of course, the community midwife was going in as well.'

That added up to two visits a week. No wonder Eliza wasn't able to manage. Initially, I thought, she needed a daily visit at home.

'Well,' I said, 'I think they'll be ready to have Susan at home by the end of the week, but I think she'll need to be visited every day for a bit. In the end, I think they will manage fine.'

'We've had several discussions about this and we've decided that, when Susan comes out, she should go into care. Eliza can take her home, once the care home think she can cope.'

'Where's the care home?'

She named a home fifty miles away.

'That won't work,' I said. 'The parents don't drive and it'll take hours for Eliza to get there and back each day. Much simpler to provide support at home. It wouldn't take a lot of time each day and it'll get less as Eliza manages better.'

'I'm sorry,' she said. 'We've decided. Let me know when Eliza's fit to be discharged and I'll make the arrangements.'

'Well, she could go today, if that's the case, but you'll have to sign a form saying that you are taking her out of hospital against medical advice.'

There was a horrified pause. I knew that social services had the right to make this decision, but it was the only way I could think of to make them pause. I knew they wouldn't want to expose themselves by doing this.

'Let me talk to my colleagues,' she said, to buy time.

Over the next five days I received regular calls from increasingly senior social services managers, asking me to relent, but I refused. Eventually, the Director of Social Services called, someone I knew quite well.

'Hello, David, what can I do for you?' I said, knowing perfectly well what he'd called about.

'All right, you win,' he said. 'Give us a couple of days to

arrange support and Susan can go home with her parents.'

'Great,' I said, relieved.

Susan went home and Eliza, with John, had daily support for about six months. I heard later that all had gone well for quite a while, but then Eliza and John had separated and, eventually, Susan was brought up by her paternal granny. You can't win them all.

12.

Sometimes Organic, Sometimes Not

Whenever the topic of attention deficit hyperactivity disorder (ADHD) comes up, there is always a fierce debate. Much of it centres around what is often seen as the inappropriate use of drugs to manage the condition. These heated discussions are often rather poorly informed, because not many understand how broad the spectrum of young people with ADHD is.

WILFRED
Wilfred James was a good example of the severe end of the spectrum. When I first met him, he was about six years old and completely uncontrollable. He would sleep at night, but, once up, he was in constant movement all day, never settling to one task or interest for more than a few seconds, perhaps thirty at the most. His mother was driven to distraction and the school completely unable to cope with him.

I assessed him in my clinic, with considerable difficulty, and felt that he fitted the criteria for ADHD very well. He was clearly hyperactive, never sitting still for long. He was extremely inattentive, making lots of mistakes. However, even while rushing about, he could sometimes carry on talking about a subject that interested him, like space flight. He talked a lot, often ceaselessly, interrupting others often.

I thought he needed treatment with Ritalin, chemical name methylphenidate, urgently. This is THE drug that some parents think is overused. I think they are often right, but in children like Wilfred, it can be magical. It's actually a stimulant, working as a dopamine reuptake inhibitor. In patients like Wilfred, it has a paradoxical effect, slowing them down. If you see this response, it shows firstly that you've made the right diagnosis and secondly, underlines that there is a basic neurochemical abnormality.

It took quite a long time and a higher than usual dose of methylphenidate to get Wilfred suitable managed. In order to get his dose as low as was feasible for him to lead a reasonably normal life, he came into the ward.

It was fascinating to watch him in the morning. The nursing staff always caught him to give him his Ritalin as he woke up because, if they didn't, he would leap out of bed. He did that anyway and would run round and round the central ward block, which was about 60 ft square, getting slower and slower as his medicine kicked in. Eventually, he was reasonably slow and would sit down for breakfast.

He had more doses during the day and went to bed fairly quietly, always sleeping well, thank goodness. We eventually worked out a regime that suited him and that Mrs James could manage at home. Wilfred had a sister three years younger, Virginia, so Mrs James had plenty on her hands.

Everything went well for about six years. We increased the dose as he grew and he was doing well at school. I wasn't seeing him very often, twice a year, because his ADHD was under control. Then Mrs James rang up my wonderful secretary, Gill. All my patients knew her well and trusted her. She worked with me for twenty-six years and at my hospital for over forty years, by the time she retired.

'Oh Gill, please can you fix it for me to see Dr Stern soon? We've got a problem.'

'What's wrong?' said Gill, solicitously.

'It's a bit complicated, but they're threatening to stop his treatment!' Mrs James said, almost crying.

'Who is?' asked Gill.

'It's some new community doctor, I can't remember his name.'

'All right, I will fit you in somewhere. Monday all right?'

'Thanks, that's great.'

When I met Wilfred and Betty James in the clinic, he was fine. The Ritalin hadn't yet been stopped. It turned out that there was a new Senior Registrar in Community Paediatrics who had been reviewing a number of patients. Eventually, he met Wilfred and his mother.

'He said that Wilfred's treatment was out of date. That lots of children with ADHD didn't need any drugs and that he thought he could be managed by CBT, whatever that is.'

'That's cognitive behavioural therapy. CBT is very good for

the right patients. I know that Wilfred isn't one of them. Don't worry, I'll have a talk with him.'

I met Dr Bannerjee in my office. He started straight in.

'I don't think it's good modern therapy to give ADHD patients methylphenidate. Most of them don't need any drugs,' he stated firmly.

'Quite true,' I agreed, to his surprise. 'I don't use it very often. Wilfred needs it, though. Have you read his hospital notes?'

'No, I haven't. May I?'

'Of course,' I said and left him to read them for twenty minutes. They were quite extensive!

'What do you think?' I asked him.

'I can see that he needed Ritalin when he was younger, but how do you know he still does?' he asked, reasonably.

'Because, as he grows, he becomes more and more hyperactive. As you can see from his notes, I've had to increase the dose over the years, slowly.'

'Yes, but he's on a very large dose, compared to other children with ADHD.'

'I know, because he needs it.'

'Well, I'd like to try him off treatment for a trial period.'

'I'd advise strongly against it,' I counselled. 'I think Mrs James' life will become intolerable.'

We agreed to differ. I wrote to the Consultant in Community Medicine recommending that, under no circumstances should they stop his treatment. For a month, I heard nothing. Then Mrs James came rushing into my clinic with her daughter and

Wilfred. He did sit down but continually shifted around, here, there and everywhere.

'They had a big meeting and invited me. They said they were going to stop his treatment and see what happened. I pleaded with them not to, but they did anyway. Wilfred is out of control; the school have excluded him. And now Virginia's starting to behave like him too.'

This sort of imitative behaviour in siblings is not unknown.

'I suspect she's copying Wilfred. Let's ignore them and start his treatment again. You can get it from the children's pharmacy here for the moment, so we can bypass them.'

We did so. It took us nearly four months to help Wilfred to get back to where he was. During that time, the community doctors decided to take action against what we were doing and the case went to a tribunal. I couldn't find the time to attend, but I sent a long report.

Mrs James came to my clinic afterwards, I knew it was good news, because she was wearing a big smile.

'What happened?' I asked.

'The judge listened to their case. It went on a long time and they quoted lots of references. They came to the end. "What about this?" said the judge, waving your report. They said that they didn't think it was relevant. "Why not?" he asked. They said it was just a description of how Wilfred's problem had developed over the years. "Exactly," said the judge. "It's quite clear from Dr Stern's report that Wilfred needs methylphenidate treatment and that, if he doesn't have it, his life and that of his family is intolerable. Case dismissed!"'

I'm afraid that none of this would have happened had the doctors in this case been prepared to trust my experience, instead of listening to their own prejudices.

PATRICK

Sometimes the way in which children react to a change in circumstances can be startling. Patrick was fourteen when his mother, Celia Stewart, brought him to my clinic. He had been referred by his GP, who told me that, from being a pleasant and capable boy, he had become difficult to manage.

'He doesn't seem to be the same boy he used to be,' said Mrs Stewart, while Patrick sat glowering at her. He obviously didn't want to be here.

'He was always so helpful, now he won't do anything for me. He sits in his bedroom all the time, except when he's at school. And he's been truanting from school, too. Twice in the last month.'

'Is that so?' I asked Patrick.

'Suppose.'

'What's the problem?' I asked him.

'Dunno.'

I took the rest of the story. His birth and past history was normal, but the family history was interesting. When Patrick was eight, his father had died suddenly, leaving Celia and her three children on their own. At the time, Patrick's sister Susan was seven and the youngest brother, Peter, was five, so they were all at school.

'Patrick was a real help then. I went to work, so my mother came to look after the children when I wasn't able to be there.

But she's not very fit and Patrick did everything to help to make the house run smoothly. Now he's changed so much!'

'Has anything changed at home?'

'Not really, but I've got a new partner, Steven. He's fitting in really well.'

I glanced at Patrick. He looked away.

'Does he get on with Patrick?' I asked. He snorted.

'I think so, but they don't talk much.'

'Have you noticed any other odd incidents?'

'Well, yes. May I speak to you in private?'

We moved into a clinic room with the door partly closed.

'I lost a screwdriver a week or so ago. I needed it to change a plug. Then I noticed that Patrick was walking oddly. After a bit of a set-to, I found that he's stuck it down the front of his trousers!'

By now, the situation was clear. For several years, Patrick had been acting as the quasi-father figure in the family. Now he was being displaced by Steven and his role had changed. He didn't know how to fit into the new family structure and resented losing his position as his mother's 'partner'.

I discussed this, first with Celia and then together with Patrick. He tried to look disinterested, in the way adolescents often do.

'We can do quite a lot to make things easier. I know it would help for Patrick to be able to talk through his new family situation and how he feels about it with someone else. Our Clinical Psychologist, Melanie, would be exactly the right person to meet. Shall I set that up for you, Patrick?' I half-expected him to say 'No', but he just shrugged. I took that as assent.

Melanie told me it took about a month to get Patrick to open up but, once he could verbalise his feelings, things began to fall into place. After six months, everything settled down.

MICHAEL AND MICAH

Occasionally I might be asked to see the child of a colleague. This could mean arranging a special consultation, if there were clashes in our clinic appointments. One such occurred when I was asked to see the three-year-old twin sons of a consultant neurologist. He and his wife were concerned about their behaviour and their learning. They were not yet speaking and they found managing them very difficult.

I met them early one afternoon in our children's clinic. As there was no other scheduled clinic that day, we were the only people there: Archie Stirling and his wife Jennifer, plus Micah and Michael.

Archie, Jennifer and I sat in a clinic room while the children played outside. We left the door open, to keep an eye on them, as there was no clinic nurse present.

I started to take a history, but we were frequently distracted by the behaviour of the two boys. To say that their play was unstructured would be putting it mildly. They played quite independently and managed to destroy everything that could be broken, torn up or otherwise made unusable.

'This is what they are like at home,' said Jennifer. 'We have to try to confine them to safe spaces, which seems to work, but they simply don't listen. We wonder whether they're deaf, but they do react appropriately to sound.'

'I tested their hearing some time ago,' said Archie. 'I think it's quite normal.'

At intervals, I took a history. They were a Jewish family, but completely unrelated, so recessive genetic disorders seemed unlikely. There was a sister, now eleven years old, who was doing well at school.

'She did have communication problems when she was younger, but she grew out of them by the time she was four or five, more or less. She's fine now.'

'What sort of problems?'

'Well, a bit like this,' said Jennifer. 'But much less marked.'

Apart from it being a twin pregnancy, the rest of the history was unremarkable. Although I was fairly sure of the diagnosis now, it was time to look at them.

'Come here, Michael,' said Archie. He ignored the summons. Archie went out and picked him up, sitting him on his lap. I knelt in from of him.

'Hello, Michael,' I said. He looked straight through me. I might just as well have been a gatepost. The diagnosis was clear.

'You know what's wrong with them, Archie, don't you?'

'No, that's why I asked you to see them.'

It's a truism that it is very hard to pick up on what's wrong with your own children, however expert you are and Archie was a nationally renowned neurologist.

'They are both autistic and, I would say, well along the spectrum to the more severe end.'

Archie looked amazed and then relaxed.

'Of course, it's quite obvious now. I can't think why I didn't realise it, though we had an inkling.'

'When it's under your nose and you see it developing day by day, it's much harder to pick up on,' I said.

'Well, what do we do now?'

'You need lots of specifically trained educational input, every day, coming into the house to go through a programme of training that's has been shown to be highly beneficial. I'm sure we can set this up and they can be helped. Once the diagnosis has been made, the local authority has a duty to provide this for them. It can take a while to put in place, because they move rather slowly, but I will write supportive letters and we'll start to pressurise them.'

'Do you think Angela is autistic as well?' asked Jennifer.

'Obviously I don't know but, from your description it's quite likely. Autism does run in families in about 20–30 per cent of cases. It's one reason why some parents became convinced that MMR was responsible, because they might have two or three children with it and it appears around the second year of life. That it might be genetic seems to be ignored by them.'

The family went off home and I started writing to their local authority. As usual, it took a while for me to get a response and, to begin with, it wasn't encouraging. I was surprised, therefore, when three months later the Stirlings came back to the clinic and Archie told me everything was in place. They had a team of teachers coming in and following the programme and the boys were starting to respond.

'How did you manage that?' I asked.

Archie reached into his bag and pulled out a ring-binder that had 5 cm thick of documents in it.

'I researched the literature and came up with lots of papers supporting the need for this therapy,' he said. 'I gave it to them and it seemed to do the trick!'

I went through them briefly. It was a brilliantly edited collection of the relevant peer reviewed and published literature on the management of children with autism. Naturally, I wasn't surprised. Archie was an outstanding clinical neurologist and this was easy for him to do.

'Please may I have a copy?' I asked, thinking it would be incredible useful for other patients of mine.

'I knew you'd ask for it. This *is* a copy for you!'

I was very grateful. After that, I used the folder several times. It only failed once. By that time, unbeknownst to me, local authorities had altered their guideline on caring for autistic children.

About a year before I retired, I picked up another child with autism. As usual, I wrote to the local authority asking for support for him. Six months later, the parents rang me.

'Nothing's happened,' the mother said.

'Why not?'

'I've been told that you're not allowed to make a diagnosis of autism. He's got to be seen by someone at Guy's Hospital.'

I knew at once who that was. A colleague of mine at Guy's was and still is the national authority on autism. Apparently, there had been an agreement that every case in the south-east of England had to be confirmed by her. I was not happy!

I rang her up and she was equally outraged. She didn't even know about this agreement between local authorities. She wrote to every relevant local authority to say 'If Colin Stern makes a diagnosis of autism, then you must accept it.' I thought that was very kind and helpful of her.

The boy got his treatment in place soon afterwards.

GERALDINE

Geraldine was referred urgently by her GP. Dr Smithers telephoned to ask whether I could see her that morning. Apparently, her mother, Sheila Dampier, had brought her to the surgery, because twelve-year-old Geraldine was having difficulty breathing. She identified stridor, which is noisy breathing on breathing *in* and raises the possibility of inflammation of the larynx, causing partial obstruction to the airway. This can be a medical emergency, so I wondered why Dr Smithers hadn't sent her straight to Children's A&E.

'Well, she said. 'There's something a bit odd about it. The stridor is very loud, but Geraldine doesn't have a temperature and seems untroubled. Mrs Dampier told me she had it for several days now, but, because her daughter was so well, she didn't worry too much about it, thinking it was just mild laryngitis. As it wasn't showing any sign of going away, she thought I'd better see her. I really don't know what's going on.'

As I was already in my clinic, I suggested she came in that morning and I would squeeze her in somehow. The Clinic Sister and the Clerk would be cross with me, but that couldn't be helped.

In due course, Geraldine and Sheila Dampier arrived, accompanied by Delilah, the Clinic Clerk.

'I've registered her and given you a temporary set of notes. That'll have to do,' Delilah said, reprovingly.

'Thank you very much, Delilah, I'm sorry to have caused you all this trouble. Don't worry, Gill will sort it out later.'

All this time, the Dampiers were sitting there, but not quietly: Geraldine was making quite a loud noise when she breathed in, rather like a coarse 'whoop'. She wasn't in respiratory distress and smiled easily. Odd, I thought.

'When did this begin?'

'Last Thursday,' said Mrs Dampier. That was four days earlier.

'She hasn't had any fever, cough or sore throat?'

'Nothing like that.'

'You haven't swallowed and choked on anything?' I asked Geraldine.

She shook her head between 'whoops'.

I examined her. I didn't get a good look in her throat, as she found this too distressing. however, she was otherwise perfectly normal and there were no abnormal chest signs other than the stridor.

'Does she make this noise all the time?' I asked.

'Only during the daytime.'

Aha!

'So she is absolutely fine at night.'

'Yes, she's been sleeping just as normal. That's one reason why I wasn't too worried to begin with.'

As Geraldine's stridor wasn't present when she was asleep,

this had to be hysterical stridor.

'Has everything been quite normal at home?'

'Oh yes, and she's been doing well at school, she loves it.'

'Nothing has changed at all?'

'No, apart from Harry.'

'Who's Harry?'

'He's about to be my husband. We've been together for a few months and he moved in ten days ago. We're getting married in a month or two, when we can get the money together. We want a proper celebration.'

'Are you looking forward to this, Geraldine?'

A shrug.

'Do Harry and Geraldine get on all right?'

'I think so,' said Mrs Dampier. 'He's a very quiet man and has been trying his best to get to know the children.' Geraldine had a brother called Dick, who was ten.

I bit the bullet.

'Geraldine has what we would call hysterical stridor. This is usually the result of some stress and, in her case, the change in her family structure may be the reason. Obviously, I don't know that for sure. In Geraldine's case, although the stridor isn't dangerous, it will impair her lifestyle, it'll make it difficult to go to school. I suggest that she come into hospital for a day or two, so that I can introduce her to our psychologist Laura, who will work with her to identify the reason for the stridor and start some therapy. With good luck, we'll stop the sound fairly quickly.'

I was being a bit optimistic. Sometimes it can take a long time to bring this sort of symptom under control. The other reason for bringing her in is obvious. I needed to make sure that there wasn't anything more sinister behind Geraldine's stridor and her relationship with Harry.

Geraldine came in for three days. We were lucky. Harry turned out to be a very pleasant and appropriate stepfather. Geraldine had been acting as a surrogate second parent to her brother, following his sudden departure two years before. The change in family dynamics had unsettled her to the extent that she developed the stridor. Once she had talked all this though with Laura, the stridor vanished.

A triumph for 'talking therapies'.

ANTHONY

Anthony was fourteen years old. His mother, Victoria Johnstone, was worried about his heart. The family doctor, Martin Smith, wrote that she had brought him to see her several times, to say that he seemed breathless and had been complaining of palpitations in his chest. He had taken a good look at him on each visit, but not found anything wrong. Every time she came with him, Mrs Johnstone was becoming more anxious and so he asked me to see Anthony.

I took a history from his mother. She was a thin Afro-Caribbean lady who was clearly under stress. One issue of concern she had was that five relatives had passed away after having heart problems.

'It run in the family, doctor,' she said, wringing her hands. 'Both his great-uncles and his grandfather died from a heart problem, as well as me mother and she was only in her late thirties. We have weak hearts,' she pronounced.

'What do you notice wrong?' I asked Anthony.

He looked a bit lost.

'When Anthony come home from school, he always having trouble catching his breath. He sit down at the table and, after a while, his breathing settle. When I point it out to him, he just say that he running from the bus stop.' Anthony nodded. 'But he the same when he come from playing in the park, football with friends. Sometime I can see his heart pumping away and once he say he can feel it. I think he must have something wrong with it. He need an X-ray or something.'

'Let me have a look at you.'

I spent a while checking Anthony out. He was quite normal and healthy. His blood pressure was normal, his pulse rate was normal, there were no heart murmurs, his heart wasn't enlarged and his chest completely clear. His height and weight were normal for his age. He was well through the onset of puberty.

I decided, in view of Mrs Johnstone's concern, that I needed to carry out some investigations. After so many consultations, I didn't think I could allay them just by saying he was fine.

'I can arrange for Anthony to have a chest X-ray and an electrocardiograph (ECG) this morning and, I hope, we can do this now and I will see you with the results at the end of this clinic. That will give me lots of information about how his heart is working. The tests aren't painful and of very low risk. Will that be all right with you both?'

'Yes, thank you doctor,' said Victoria. Anthony nodded in reluctant agreement.

Off they went. I met them again about two hours later. They were carrying the chest X-ray folder and an envelope containing his ECG. I put his chest X-ray on the light box.

'There's your heart, Anthony, and these are your lungs. Your heart is the size it ought to be and there's nothing unusual about its shape. Yours lungs are healthy too. Here's the report, and you can see the radiologist thought it was entirely normal.'

I spread out the ECG on the desk.

'These are the electrical waves produced by your heart contracting. This pattern here is produced when your heart contracts and relaxes. This is the "P" wave, made when the atria, the little chambers at the top of the heart, contract. They're normal and the space between that and what we call the QRS complex is fine. The QRS complex is normal too. It shows that your heart is functioning exactly as it should.'

I sat back and thought. I decided to follow a hunch.

'Now you know that Anthony's heart and its function are normal, do you think you could tell me what the real problem you have is?'

There was a pause. Victoria looked at me blankly for a moment, then she burst in floods of tears. I handed her a box of tissues and waited.

'It's me stepmother,' she said. 'She passed away three weeks ago and I want to go to her funeral.'

This was puzzling. 'What's stopping you?'

'Me sister,' she said, weeping again.

It turned out that Victoria's mother, her only parent, had died when Victoria was only eight years old. She had been adopted by another family. This adoption had been extremely successful, Victoria had been well cared for and very happy. She grew up with her stepmother's daughter, who was two years older than her. The parents were unable to have any more children and the two girls enjoyed a happy childhood.

Victoria left school and worked in a shop, where she met her husband Lewis. He was still around and they were very happy. They had three children, of which Anthony was the eldest.

About eight years ago, the two sisters had fallen out over some quite trivial matter. They had not spoken since.

When Victoria's stepmother had died, she had asked to go to the funeral. As her adoption had never been formalised, she had no legal membership of the family, in spite of living in it for ten years. Her sister refused to allow her to come to the funeral and would not answer the phone to her.

Victoria's complaints about Anthony were her way of expressing her grief and frustration.

I thought this needed to be dealt with urgently, as her stepmother's funeral was to be held soon.

'Do you have your sister's telephone number?' I asked.

'Yes.'

'Please may I have it?'

I took the number and asked Victoria and Anthony to go and have some lunch, while I finished my clinic. I arranged to meet them later in my office.

I telephoned Samantha, Victoria's stepsister. When I said what it was about, she almost put the phone down on me.

'That woman! I won't have her near Mum.'

Eventually, I was able to put the situation to her quietly. She calmed down. After a while, she became more understanding.

'All right,' she said eventually, 'She can come. I had no idea that it would cause all this trouble. I suppose it's about time we got over it.'

Whatever 'it' was, I never discovered.

Victoria was relieved and happy. Some weeks later I had a card from her. Samantha and Victoria had made it up and their families were meeting again. Anthony was still as fit as a fiddle.

JULIAN

An old acquaintance from medical school was principal in a large group practice in an affluent suburb. He persuaded me to run a monthly paediatric clinic in his practice, which I did for about five years. Julian was one of several interesting patients that I met at this time.

Julian's mother, Delia, was a local businesswoman with her own company. Her husband, Tom Daniels, also had his own company, in a different field. They had met at university and been together ever since.

Their GP, Dr Simon Ho, asked me to see them because Delia was very worried that Julian might have autism. This was at a time when a lot of false information was circulating about links between MMR immunisation and autism, although this was not the link here, because Julian was only six months old!

Simon was an outstandingly able GP, so I said to him that this seemed an odd referral.

'Yes,' he said. 'The whole thing is rather odd. Delia has

raised the same concern with various professionals: professors of obstetrics, your old friend David and another professor of neonatology. They have all tried to reassure her without any effect.'

'If they can't do so, I think it's unlikely that I'll be able to,' I protested.

'Well,' he replied. 'See her and Julian and have a go. You never know.'

In due course, Delia, Tom and Julian appeared in the clinic. I was intrigued by her anxiety about autism, because, at six months, there wasn't any way I would be able to say that Julian *didn't* have it, however unlikely it might seem.

I decided to start from scratch.

'Dr Ho tells me that you are worried that Julian might be autistic.'

'Yes,' said Delia. 'I can't stop worrying about it.'

'Do you have relations that have autism, then?'

'Not that we know of.'

'So, how do you know about the condition then?'

'I suppose it goes back to my time at university. I did a combined honours course in biological sciences and, as my project, worked with a group of autistic children, on their psychosocial interactions within and outside their families. I learned a lot doing it, but I also was aware of how difficult life within their families could be.'

'Do you think that's why you became worried about Julian?'

'Not exactly. When I became pregnant, I studied several books giving advice to new mothers on how best to look after yourself and your baby during pregnancy and early childhood. One thing I learned was what made a good diet for a pregnant mum. I got the idea that liver was good for you, so for the first couple of months I ate lots of liver. Then I found out that too much liver can damage the developing fetus, particularly the brain, and that this might lead to autism. That's what made me so scared.'

'It's made it hard for her to sleep at night,' said Tom. 'Not that we sleep much anyway,' he continued, laughing as he looked at Julian, who was asleep.

'I was booked to have Julian at a private hospital and had several discussions with my consultant, who said it wasn't his area of expertise; I needed to speak with their paediatrician,' said Delia. 'I met him, both before and after Julian was born and he was very reassuring, saying that Julian didn't have anything to suggest autism, but I have gone on worrying. We took him to a professor of paediatric neurology, who said the same, but I am still worried.'

'Is there anything about Julian that makes you feel he is autistic?' I asked.

'Yes,' Delia said. 'He won't look at me, whatever I do. I am sure this is a reflection of the lack of personal interaction that's typical of autistic children.' It seemed as though she had already made the diagnosis.

At this moment, Julian woke up. It was a good time to examine him. He was an entirely healthy six-month-old baby boy.

I thought it was important to see whether I could get him to look at me and, more importantly, Delia. I stood with my face to the window, holding Julian in front of me. I had Delia on my right shoulder and Tom at my left. Julian fixed his eyes firmly on my face and, after a pause, smiled. Delia was surprised. I moved him so that first, he looked at Delia and then at Tom. Goodness they were happy!

'Well,' I said. 'I'm afraid that doesn't tell us much, except that he is very happy to see you, which is the first stage of interacting with you. However, I can't tell you whether or not he has autism. He's much too young.'

Luckily, this turned out to be exactly what Delia Daniels needed to hear.

'I know,' she said. 'They keep trying to tell me there's nothing wrong with him, but I know that they can't tell yet. That's half the problem.'

'It'll be a year or two before we can be certain,' I said. 'In the meantime, it's best not to worry too much about it, because it's very important that you treat him as though he is entirely normal. Difficult, I know, but do your best.'

'Would you go on seeing him from time to time?' said Delia.

'Of course. Why don't we meet every six months or so, and we'll see how he gets on.'

They agreed.

At the next visit, Delia Daniels said, 'He never looks at me! I'm sure it's a sign.' Julian was not quite walking, but he watched and babbled at me and then his parents.

'Why does he always look at *you*?' Delia complained. She was clearly paranoid about the likelihood of autism. I was becoming anxious.

Throughout all this, Tom Daniels was a model husband. He never challenged her, acted in the most encouraging way and he was incredibly supportive. This proved crucial because, after their third clinic appointment, Mrs Daniels had a complete mental breakdown and was admitted for inpatient care to a nearby psychiatric unit. Tom looked after Julian, both his and her businesses and supported her as well. Truly a multi-tasking husband.

Eventually, Delia was discharged home, much improved. I met them again twice. The second time, Delia brought her new baby daughter, Lydia, with her.

'I can understand now how it was I became so anxious about Julian. It became an unhealthy obsession and took over my life. Thinking about it now sends shivers down my spine.'

Julian was by then a happy five-year-old and loved his little sister. All was well in the end.

13.

Don't Swallow It!

LUCAS

Lucas was a twelve-year-old boy who came to our Children's A&E with a history of nausea, diarrhoea and vomiting. He had also brought up a small amount of blood. His symptoms had begun during the night, so his mother, Lydia Mortimer, had given him a proprietary preparation, designed for gastroenteritis. By morning, he was still unwell and she began to think he was becoming a bit sleepy and confused, so brought him in.

He was assessed by our A&E team, who agreed with her diagnosis, but thought he was a bit dry. As he had been vomiting as well, they started intravenous fluids and admitted him. We met Lucas and his mother on our ward round.

'He's a bit better now he's got some liquids in him,' said Mrs Mortimer. 'But, he still feels sick, don't you, Lucas?'

Lucas gave a feeble nod. He certainly looked rather sleepy.

'What did you eat yesterday?' I asked Lucas. He didn't seem to understand what I was saying.

'He's a bit confused,' said Lydia. 'He had his usual cereal for breakfast, same as the rest of us. Lunch at school, but I don't know what that was, 'cos he can't seem to remember. I rang the school and there've been no other reports of children being unwell. In the evening we all had a steak and kidney pie that I'd made, with veg, and he had some ice cream, as Celia his sister did. She's fine.'

'Is that all Lucas?' I asked again. He seemed to agree.

'Anyone he's been in contact with been unwell, or had a fever or sore throat?'

'Not that we have been able to discover.'

'Has he had any other problems?'

'Only toothache yesterday evening, but I gave him something for that.'

'What did you give him?'

'Some oil of cloves. Lucas likes it, because he says it really helps. I put some on his tooth with a cotton bud and a teaspoon, but he swallowed the lot! Said it tasted nice.'

Oh dear. I thought I knew what had happened here. I examined him and couldn't find any evidence of infection.

'Lucas, I think you've fallen foul of my old friend Eugene,' I said.

'Who's he?' asked Mrs Mortimer.

'Well, actually it's a chemical called eugenol, but I always think of him as Eugene. It's one of the agents in oil of cloves. The trouble is that it's quite toxic in fairly small doses. That's why you should only dab a little on the painful tooth. It works very well, though.'

'Can you do anything about it?'

'Well, we can, but it may be a bit too late,' I said, injudiciously.

'Lucas ingested it rather too long ago, but we'll give him the usual treatment. He's still fairly well, but we'll check him over and make sure. He'll need to stay here for a few days.'

We continued his fluids, gave him some activated charcoal and checked his liver function, which, fortunately, was normal. Liver damage is a higher risk in children with eugenol poisoning.

His conscious level was definitely affected and he took three or four days to recover enough to go home.

Lots of families keep oil of cloves in the bathroom cabinet, but not many know that it can be dangerous.

ABRAHAM

Abraham was admitted at a year of age, because of unexplained anaemia. He was born following a normal pregnancy and had been a happy baby. His GP said that, over the last few weeks he had become rather irritable, being difficult to settle down. His mother had brought him to the surgery, where Dr Adamski had noticed that he looked anaemic, so referred him to my clinic.

Susannah Jacobs brought in Abraham, her son. He was grizzling a little.

'He doesn't seem very happy this morning,' she said. 'He's been like this, on and off, for a few weeks. Nothing seems to pacify him. We haven't been getting much sleep,' she added, with a sigh.

I took a history. There was nothing out of the ordinary about it. I examined him. He did look to be clinically anaemic, but all babies can look a bit anaemic at this age. This, however, seemed more than that. I could hear a few fine crackles at his lung bases.

'He seems a bit chesty,' I said.

'Yes, he's had a slight cough for a few days.'

'It would be a good idea to sort this out this morning,' I said. 'We'll arrange some investigations and see you with the results at the end of the clinic.'

We were fortunate that, for basic investigations, we could obtain rapid results, which saved both time and the need to admit a child unnecessarily. I wrote some forms out for straightforward blood tests and a chest X-ray. They came back at the end of the clinic.

As it happened, I put the X-ray up on the box first. The report said that his chest was clear. Alerted, I took a closer look at it. I turned to my SHO, Dr McIntyre.

'What do you think of that?'

He took a careful look. 'As the report says, his lungs are clear and his heart look normal.'

'What about his humeri?' These are the long bones in the upper arms, which were shown on the chest X-Ray.'

'Oh,' he said. 'They each have a denser line at the epiphyses. What is it?'

'I think they are lead lines,' I replied. 'Let's have a look at his blood count.'

Sure enough, he had an iron deficiency type anaemia and there was basophilic stippling in his red blood cells. The report suggested he might have lead poisoning. I should have looked at it first!

'I'm afraid we will need to admit Abraham for a little while. His tests suggest that he has lead poisoning, though we'll need to do another test to confirm it. It explains all his symptoms, including his irritability. Have you any idea how he might have eaten it?'

'No idea at all,' said Mrs Jacobs. 'So far as I know, he's only eaten his food.'

'What sort of house do you live in?'

'It's a modern apartment, built about five years ago.' It couldn't be lead pipes, then.

'Have you ever found him with scraps of anything with him, in his buggy or his cot?'

'Not in his buggy. In his cot, yes. There have been bits of the paint from the wooden bars, because he keeps chewing on them. It's a family heirloom, it's been used by several generations. I've been meaning to get it repainted, once Abraham grows out of it.'

'When was it last painted?'

'A long time ago, probably before the war. My mother wanted it just as my grandmother had left it.'

There was the cause. Lead paint was still being used at that time, though it is illegal to make it now. We sent a community team to the flat to check. Sure enough, the cot had lead paint.

Abraham came into hospital, his level of blood lead was high. We managed to remove most of it, using intravenous calcium EDTA, a chelation agent which latches onto the lead, so that it can be excreted.

He did well.

ASHALINA

Ashalina was a baby of fifteen months. Her mother had taken her to her family doctor because, for the last few days, Amina Gamal, Ashalina's mother, had noticed that her baby was more floppy than before and that she didn't seem to like the light. Dr O'Sullivan thought she was rather red-faced, but couldn't find any evidence of fever or infection. He asked me to see her.

'I don't know what's wrong,' Mrs Gamal wailed. 'I try to soothe her, but nothing helps.' She spoke no English, but this was Panya Mohammed the interpreter's version.

'That's why you've come. We'll do our best to find out what's going on.'

The Gamals had come to the UK from Egypt, when her husband, an economist, was recruited to join their embassy in London. He brought his wife and their five children, of whom Ashalina was the youngest. The other four, aged ten, eight, seven and five, were all in English school.

'When did you notice that Ashalina's behaviour changed?' I asked.

'Last week. She was a bit more floppy', translated Panya.

'Anything else?' I waited while there was a hurried conversation.

'No,' came the surprisingly short answer.

Mrs Gamal had come with a history provided by her husband, which saved me some time. The other children, two girls and two boys, were all healthy. He didn't know of any family illnesses. They had also brought Amina's mother with them to England, to help with the children.

'What does your mother do to help you?' I asked.

There was another, rather longer discussion.

'She helps me look after the children. Also, I am learning English, so she cares for Ashalina when I go for lessons.'

'How often is that?'

'Every weekday just now. I have been going since just after we arrived, two months ago.'

'So, you must be speaking English better now,' I hazarded.

She gave a weak smile. 'I try,' she said, hesitantly. 'Soon I am all right in English. Better Panya come with me today.'

'Yes, it's a good thing. Medicine can be a bit complicated.' She smiled and Panya translated for her.

I had a look at Ashalina, who needed to be prised away from Mrs Gamal and unwrapped from her almost completely enveloping shawls first.

She was a red-faced baby who instinctively turned from the light. Definitely photophobia, but nothing to suggest a fever or meningism. Her hands and feet were very red too. She was also hypotonic – floppier than normal.

There was some greyish dried powder at the corner of her mouth.

'What's this?' I asked, pointing it out. Another discussion between Panya and Amina.

'It's what my mother gave her.'

'What for?' More discussion.

'Ashalina has been later than her brothers and sisters to produce her teeth. Amina's mother says she is rubbing her gums and needs help to breed them. She has been giving her something to ease her gums.'

The idea that teething is painful is ancient. Children become fussier when teeth are about to come through and they have been shown to have more minor infections. I think this is just because everything gets put in the mouth at that age, so they pick up any bug that's around. Teething powders were given for this, but were discontinued after the Second World War in the UK.

'What did she give her?'

'It's a family remedy she brought from Egypt.'

'Did the other children have it too?'

'No, because Amina was giving all the care to them as babies in Egypt. Her mother looked after the older children then.'

I knew already that Ashalina had acrodynia, otherwise known as Pink Disease, on account of the redness of the face, hands and feet. It is caused by mercury poisoning, which used to be found in teething powders and in other things, such as cosmetics. Mercury is a highly poisonous heavy metal and Ashalina needed to have it removed from her body quickly.

'I think the teething powder is the cause of the problem,' I said. 'We need to admit Ashalina to the children's ward, check her blood and do some other tests, then start her on a medicine to get the mercury out of her body.'

Amina was very distressed at this news but, between us, Panya and I calmed her down.

'Don't worry, you can stay with her. Granny can look after the children, but get her to throw away her powder and tell her not to give the children anything else until it's been checked.'

Ashalina's blood level of mercury was very high. It took a week to get her level down with 2,3 dimercaptosuccinic acid, another chelating agent. She took a little longer to recover but, in the end, she recovered. So far as I know, there were no long-term effects.

14.

Death

Death in children is, fortunately, rare. Dealing with these tragic events is extremely difficult, not only for the family, but also for the medical staff, who may have been caring for the child for a long time. I was blessed with a superb team of nurses, not least by my ward sisters, one of whom became the focus of an attempt I made to impress upon my colleagues their wonderful skills.

Many years ago, the general medical staff rounds at my hospital included weeks when our paediatric team would be asked to present cases. The responsibility seemed to fall to me, rather frequently, to arrange them. On one occasion, I thought I would spend the session explaining how we dealt with these dreadful events. I planned to have a card up my sleeve.

There were three children. The first I will call William, who was eight years old. He was admitted with a history of pallor and weakness, which had been present for about a month. When I met him, he was obviously anaemic and he had an enlarged spleen. I suspected a malignancy, probably leukaemia, arranged for the appropriate tests and admitted him to our ward. Later that day. his test results were phoned through. He was suffering from myeloid leukaemia.

In those days, the prognosis for myeloid leukaemia was poor. Few children survived, although progress was being made. Indeed, Britain has always been in the forefront of the development of effective treatment for leukaemia and I am sure that we owe our steady progress to the pioneering work of Dr Humphrey Kaye, who introduced the system of clinical trials that have led to such excellent outcomes today.

I had the responsibility of breaking the news of this diagnosis to the parents. I think it is always best to do so with the whole family, including siblings, present. Fortunately, when I arrived on the ward, William had both parents in his cubicle as well as his brother aged ten and his sister, who was eight.

'I have just received the results of William's blood tests,' I began. 'They show that he has quite a lot of primitive white blood cells in his circulation. They belong to a group of white cells that we call "myeloid". They have been growing in his bone marrow rapidly and have been squeezing out the development of his red blood cells. That's why he has become so anaemic and weak.'

'Are you telling us that William has leukaemia?' asked his mother, bluntly.

'Yes,' I said. 'William has what we call acute myeloid leukaemia.'

Before I could add any more, his mother turned to William and said, 'That's it, then, you're going to die!'

I was completely gobsmacked. I couldn't think of a worse

thing to have said. Obviously we had to try to retrieve the situation. My wonderful ward sister was with us. She took charge immediately.

Sitting on the bed with her arm around William, she said, 'We've a lot to do. William will need a lot of support, because he's going to have a lot of treatment and that's going to make him feel a lot better. As you're anaemic, we will be giving you some blood first and, after that, you'll be running around here feeling a lot better. Then the haematologists, who are our blood specialists, will come and work out the best treatment to get rid of these nasty cells.'

She carried on talking to them all, in an encouraging and supportive way. After a few minutes, most people in the room, apart from her and I, had forgotten what William's mother had said. We knew that it was the shock of the diagnosis that had made her speak out.

Then there was Gabriella, a ten-year-old girl whom we had looked after for several years. She had a rare malignant tumour that was a consequence of earlier radiation treatment that had been necessary, because a benign tumour had been damaging her lower spinal cord. She had received a lot of treatment for this, although we knew that we couldn't cure her. When she came in nearing the end, we had prepared, with Gabriella and her parents, a regime that would, we hoped, allow her passing to be as gentle and peaceful as possible. Much of this was managed by the same ward sister.

Some weeks later, I received a complaint from another mother, whose daughter had been coming in monthly to have an enormous nævus (mole) removed from her back. This was done in stages, by abrading it serially with a machine rather like a sander.

'When my daughter came in last month,' she wrote, 'The nursing staff were very off-hand and unhelpful. The atmosphere was not what I had been expecting.' She continued in the same vein, ending, 'I felt I must write to complain, because it was only the previous month that I wrote to you saying how wonderful had been the care my daughter was getting.'

I checked her last admission. She had come in the day following Gabriella's death. The nursing staff, that day, were very sad and depressed and their misery had undoubtedly been transmitted into the quality of the care they were giving that day.

I used to tell this story when teaching students, asking what they thought I ought to have done. Usually, they said I should write back to the complaining mother and explain why her daughter's care had been poor that day.

'No, that's exactly what you shouldn't do,' I would respond. 'To do so would only make someone else upset as well. Just apologise and say that you're sure it won't happen again. Also share this with the rest of the team, so they know what happened.'

The third case was that of a fifteen-year-old boy, Edward. He had been a patient at another hospital, where his rare brain tumour, a pineal embryoma, had been found. It was inoperable, so he had come to us for a course of radiotherapy. This was unlikely to cure him, but would give him a significant extension of his life.

He was a confused young man. He knew that his outcome was going to be poor. At the same time, being a teenager, he wasn't sure whether he wanted to cuddle the more attractive nurses, or to be cuddled by them. My ward sister developed a support plan for him and, by the end of his treatment, he was much happier, able to enjoy what was left of his life.

I arranged for the three cases to be presented at the medical staff round by three of our SHOs. They all did excellent jobs, but I had made sure that each case only took five to ten minutes to present. After twenty minutes, they had finished, leaving another twenty-five minutes of the meeting. I went back to the podium, noticing with amusement the slightly puzzled expressions on the faces of the audience.

'Please may I introduce Sister X, who is going to explain to you how we manage death and the perceptions around it in children and their families.'

This was something of a novelty in those days. To have a nurse presenting something at a medical staff round was almost heresy! It had taken considerable persuasion to get my ward sister to do this.

She spoke for twenty minutes. I watched the audience. Several of the audience, eminent, experienced and some famous consultants, were openly in tears. There were no questions, only prolonged applause. Afterwards, several doctors came up to congratulate her. One well-known, knighted consultant came up to me.

'Colin,' he said, 'Why haven't we got nurses like that?'

'You probably have.'

15.

And So …

These cases represent some of my experiences after forty years of listening to mothers. There are so many more I could describe, though this collection contains a few of those which I thought were the more amusing, educational, dramatic or distressing.

If I have offended anyone, please believe that this was not my intention and accept my apologies. I have changed the circumstances of each case considerably, so, should anyone feel that I am describing your family, you cannot be correct. Although the clinical details are accurate and all the events did happen, the children and the families are all fictional.

Finally, I hope that most of you found this canter through the world of the general paediatrician entertaining and instructive. I hope too that some of you may have learned something that you have found useful. Thank you for putting up with me!